Ida Scudder
Missionary Doctor

Terri B. Kelly

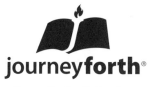

journeyforth®

Greenville, South Carolina

Library of Congress Cataloging-in Publication Data

Names: Kelly, Terri B., 1960- author.
Title: Ida Scudder : missionary doctor / Terri B. Kelly.
Description: Greenville, South Carolina : JourneyForth, [2021] |
    Audience: Ages 9-12 | Audience: Grades 4-6 | Summary: "Ida
    Scudder was the daughter of a missionary doctor. She studied to
    become one of the first lady doctors in India where she practiced
    from 1900-1960"—Provided by publisher.
Identifiers: LCCN 2021010383 | ISBN 9781646261024 (paperback) |
    ISBN 9781646261031 (ebook)
Subjects: LCSH: Scudder, Ida Sophia, 1870-1960—Juvenile literature. |
    Missionaries, Medical—India—Biography—Juvenile literature. |
    Americans—India—Biography—Juvenile literature. |
    Physicians—India—Biography—Juvenile literature. | Women
    physicians—India—Biography—Juvenile literature.
Classification: LCC R722.32.S37 K45 2021 | DDC 610.69—dc23
LC record available at https://lccn.loc.gov/2021010383

All Scripture is quoted from the King James Version.

Illustrations by Guy Porfirio
Design by Laura Davis
Page layout by Michael Boone

© 2021 BJU Press
Greenville, South Carolina 29609
JourneyForth Books is a division of BJU Press.

ISBN 978-1-64626-102-4
eISBN 978-1-64626-103-1

15 14 13 12 11 10 9 8 7 6 5 4 3 2 1

To my parents, Ernie and Marylou

CONTENTS

CHAPTER 1 1

CHAPTER 2 8

CHAPTER 3 11

CHAPTER 4 15

CHAPTER 5 20

CHAPTER 6 30

CHAPTER 7 36

CHAPTER 8 44

CHAPTER 9 49

CHAPTER 10 57

CHAPTER 11 61

CHAPTER 12 70

CHAPTER 13 77

CHAPTER 14 80

CHAPTER 15 84

CHAPTER 16 91

CHAPTER 17 98

CHAPTER 18 102

CHAPTER 19 108

CHAPTER 20 114

CHAPTER 21 121

CHAPTER 22 128

CHAPTER 23 134

CHAPTER 24 139

CHAPTER 25 148

CHAPTER 26 154

CHAPTER 27 157

CHAPTER 28 162

CHAPTER 29 165

CHAPTER 30 172

EPILOGUE 174

TERMS 177

CHAPTER 1

1889
Northfield Seminary for Girls, Massachusetts

The craving to gallop away from Northfield Seminary hit Ida Scudder like the craving for chocolate pie. Smirking, she glanced at the library door to make sure she didn't see a faculty member and untied the rope from the hitching post. Her roommates, Florence Updike and Annie Hancock, stood to the side and watched.

"What are you doing with the German professor's horse?" Annie said.

"I'm going to take this bored horse on a ride." Giggling, Ida motioned for Florence and Annie to climb in the buggy. "Hurry."

Florence stood back. "Do you know how to handle a horse and a buggy?"

"I lived on the farm in Nebraska for five years, remember?" Ida patted the seat.

Annie hesitated. "Professor Gresser's going to walk out any minute."

"Come on before anyone sees us." Ida gathered up the reins, holding them slack so she wouldn't trigger

1

the horse. "We'll take a quick ride and have the buggy back before he's finished teaching."

Annie climbed next to Ida and shook her head. "I've never done anything like this before. If we get caught—"

"We're seniors." Ida wiggled her eyebrows at the girls, knowing joy riding wasn't permitted.

Florence scooted next to Annie. "Take us on a ride, *pferd*." Florence called the German word for *horse*.

Ida shook the reins, and the horse walked down the bumpy dirt road away from campus. Golden maple trees bordered the roadside.

The horse increased its speed to a trot, crunching the leaves that blanketed the road. Annie covered her face while Florence laughed nonstop, nearly bouncing out of the seat.

A mile down the road, the horse slowed and stopped. Ida shook the reins and clicked her tongue, but the horse balked. "She won't move at all."

"Do you suppose the teacher's horse understands German commands?" Florence cupped her hand and said, "*Traben*. Trot."

The horse didn't budge.

"Yank the reins back and forth," Florence said.

"Pulling won't help." Ida jumped out of the buggy. "I wish I had a sugar cube to coax her." She rubbed the horse's mane. "Come on now, girl. Won't you take us back to school?"

Ida tried to get the horse to walk, but the horse only snorted. "We'd better hike back to campus before Miss Ford realizes we're missing." Ida tied the reins to a nearby tree.

"We're leaving the horse and buggy behind?" Annie asked.

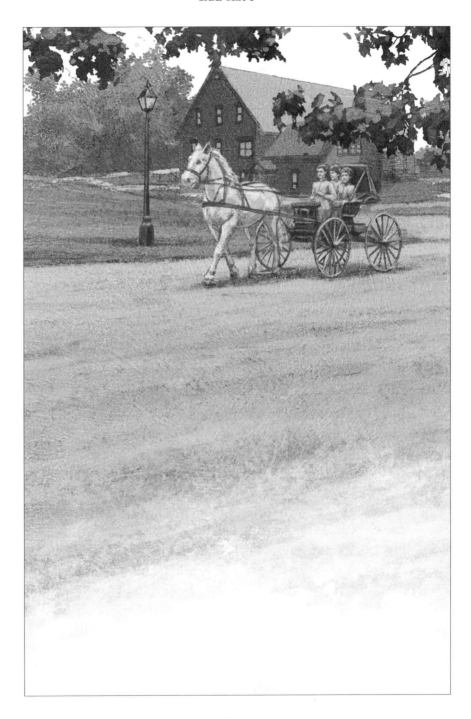

"Horses know their owner. I should have known she wouldn't take us far."

Annie gawked at Ida. "We are going to lose every senior privilege we have."

"That ride was the most fun I've had this semester." Florence laughed. "It'll be worth the loss."

Ida, Annie, and Florence ran back to campus. As the buildings came into view, they slowed to a walk before going into the dining hall. Ida sat at the far end of the long row of rectangular tables. Annie and Florence sat at the opposite end. Occasionally, Ida peeked at Florence, and both turned away to hide their smiles. Annie ignored Ida's eyes, keeping a serious face the entire meal.

The next day Miss Ford summoned Ida to her office. Ida figured she'd get more than kitchen duty for this prank. Last year Miss Ford called her to the office for giggling through chapel. The year before that she'd taken the oil stove from the school kitchen to her room and made cocoa. She'd probably miss the next dance at Mount Herman Boys' School and ruin her chances of ever having a date.

Ida tapped on the opened office door and stood statue still. Oak bookcases lined the office walls. The last time she'd been called to the office, she sidetracked the conversation by talking about growing up on the family farm in Nebraska. That tactic got Miss Ford in such a good mood, she gave Ida only one week of extra kitchen duty.

Hair pulled back in a tight bun, Miss Ford sat behind her desk and pointed to a chair. Ida sat in front of Miss Ford.

"Your escapade is not a secret. So far, Miss Scudder, your pranks are harmless. But—"

"I'm terribly sorry." Ida eyed the clock sitting on the bookshelf, hoping Miss Ford's lecture wouldn't last too long.

The headmistress smiled and lowered her voice. "I spent my share of years in boarding school too. Your grades are excellent. You are a gifted student. If only you would stop your little pranks."

Ida shifted her feet.

"I know you miss your family."

"My family is halfway around the world." Ida's tried to hide the exasperation in her voice, but mentioning family filled her with a mix of anger and sadness.

"I understand more than you know. Please," Miss Ford paused, "the girls admire you. Use your influence for good." She drew herself up. "For the horse excursion, a written apology to Professor Gresser and extra laundry duty for two—no," she flashed Ida a half-smile, "one week."

Ida sighed and closed the door. She must stop her pranks, or the school might ship her back to India with her parents. As much as she missed them, she never wanted to live in India again.

———————

Later that school year on the first day of spring at breakfast, it was Ida's turn to share a Bible verse. She waited for Miss Ford to pray before she read. She stared at the bowl of clumpy oatmeal and a tray of dry toast in front of her.

"What verse are you reading today?" Miss Ford's voice croaked.

"1 Corinthians 10:27." Ida cleared her throat. " 'Whatsoever is set before you, eat, asking no question for conscience sake.' "

Out of the corner of her eye, Ida watched the girls muffle their amusement with napkins.

"Ida Sophia Scudder." Miss Ford practically spit oat kernels with each word. "I've tolerated your pranks, but using a Bible verse to make your classmates laugh is unacceptable." The headmistress stood, the chair flying out behind her. "I expect you in my office after breakfast."

Ida, Florence, and Annie ate the rest of their breakfast in silence. From the opened windows behind the table, a breeze blew the curtains. When they finished eating, Ida led the way to the kitchen. "I might as well start washing dishes. I'm sure Miss Ford will discipline me with kitchen duty."

Ida scraped her leftover oatmeal into the trashcan. The realization of her actions pricked at her conscience. She turned to face Florence and Annie. "I used a Bible verse to support my prank. God's probably mad at me too."

"You are entertaining," Annie said. "Sometimes I wish I was bolder."

"When you grow up with five older brothers, you learn how to survive their teasing and one-up their jokes." Ida slid her hands into her front skirt pockets and stared out the window at the hills. The Connecticut River wound through the surrounding valley. Where would she go if Miss Ford expelled her?

"You best go," Annie said. "Miss Ford won't appreciate you dawdling."

Ida bit her lips and closed her eyes. "I haven't had a hug from Marmee in years. I could use one right now."

"Don't expect any hugs from Miss Ford," Florence scowled.

Ida waved goodbye. Before she turned the corner, she made a mocking face of Miss Ford for her friends.

Echoes of Florence and Annie cackling traveled through the double doors and down the steps. Ida hustled over the path beside the grassy lawn to the administration building. " 'Set a watch, O Lord, before my mouth,' " she recited. "Lord, why do I get myself in trouble like this?" Five minutes later, she took the steps to Miss Ford's third-story office.

Ida waited at the opened door.

Miss Ford stood at her desk. "Your words have more effect than you may realize."

Ida stared back. Miss Ford's tone didn't carry the usual harshness. "I'm sorry I joked with a Bible verse. My senior year isn't the year to goof around. I realize I have only two more months before graduation."

She was ready to beg. If she got kicked out, how could she go on with her plans to go to college, marry, live in a mansion, and get rich? She'd disappoint Father and Marmee if she ruined her education.

"I called you here to discuss your sarcasm, but something else has come up." She handed Ida a card. "A telegram arrived for you."

Ida's heart pounded, and her hand shook. She had received numerous letters from Father and Marmee, not telegrams.

Mother ill. Come at once.
Father

She knew it would happen. India. Dry rice fields. Bony bodies begging for food. She was being forced to return to India—the place where people got sick and . . . died.

CHAPTER 2

"**M**armee!" Tears flowed, wetting Ida's face and the collar of her dress. "She can't die."

Miss Ford took Ida's hand and led her to a chair.

"I've got to go to India." Ida pressed her hand onto her forehead, staring at the floor.

"Ida," Miss Ford said, "I can help with travel arrangements."

"I'll need money and—"

"Remember, with God nothing is impossible."

Ida covered her face with her hands. "How? Right now the situation feels impossible, and my mother—" Ida stopped. A torrent of tears gushed down her face.

"Let me discuss this with the staff. I assure you that we'll send you to India as soon as possible." Miss Ford stood and straightened her long black skirt. "Rest for a while. When you're composed, you may return to class. I'm sure your mother is going to be fine." Miss Ford's face softened.

Surely a miracle had already occurred. Ida hadn't thought Miss Ford's bony body held an ounce of compassion. Ida realized she had judged falsely. "I appreciate you," she said in a whisper.

———————

Two months later, Ida graduated from Northfield. The day after graduation Ida, Florence, and Annie trudged in silence behind the carriage driver, who carried Ida's trunk. Miss Ford stood beside the carriage door. The girls stopped and waited beside Miss Ford.

"Girls, you're so quiet and sad-faced. You look like a funeral procession." Miss Ford stepped into the carriage.

"We're all going to different places to live. Northfield's not home anymore," Annie said.

"And Ida's moving to the other side of the world." Florence dabbed her eyes with a handkerchief. "She'll never come back to America."

"I have the paperwork to prove I'm a *temporary* missionary. Four years and I'll be back." Ida patted her purse.

"I'm envious," Annie said. "What a privilege to share God's light with people who have never had the opportunity to hear it."

"Annie, I wish you were going instead of me—except I do want to see Marmee."

Miss Ford opened the carriage door and climbed inside. Ida gave Florence and Annie a quick hug and followed Miss Ford.

The carriage crossed Schell Bridge, and within thirty minutes they arrived at the Northfield Train Station. She waved goodbye to Miss Ford from the window seat in the train.

Six hours later, Ida navigated her way alone at Penn Station in New York City to meet her brother, Henry.

Ida felt confident until she stepped onto the platform. She was out of the safe cocoon of Northfield. She passed businessmen in suits and high-fashion ladies wearing fancy hats.

"Excuse me. Pardon."

How would she ever find Henry in this crowd? Ida's heart sputtered to a faster beat. She spotted a bench and made a beeline toward it. She sat and wiped the dust off her new patent leather shoes. A familiar sound cut through the hissing steam engines and calls of conductors.

Ida stopped fidgeting with her shoes, turned, and spotted someone waving a hat above the crowd.

"Idee. Idee."

A man jumped above the crowd. Her heart leapt. She recognized Henry's red hair.

"Idee," he waved his hands, "it's me, Henry. Wait."

"Henry!" Ida's voice caught in her throat. Her dress brushed against her ankles as she swerved past people toward him. A member of her family—flesh and blood Scudder. Her eyes locked onto Henry's. "Oh, I've missed you," Ida said.

Henry held her tight as they embraced. While it wasn't the hug she wanted, a hug from Henry would have to do until she reached Marmee.

CHAPTER 3

Henry stepped back and smiled. "Idee, you're all grown up."

"I'm nearly twenty, Henry."

"Look at your gorgeous golden curls." Henry cupped his hand around a ringlet dangling around her ear. "Let's transfer our trunks, and then you shall entertain me with stories of your suitors."

"Suitors?" Ida giggled. "There aren't any suitors in my life." She wrung her hands. Had she grown too old to have a suitor? She watched the porters lift the heavy trunk to the waiting carriage that would take them to the Port of New York.

Henry offered his arm for Ida and walked her toward the carriage. "How about a bag of peanuts and a cold lemonade?"

"Sounds delicious."

Henry purchased both from a vendor. "Here you are." He handed her a lemonade and tilted the bag of peanuts.

"How kind, Henry."

"This is how you should expect a suitor to treat you. Big brother is here to accompany the fine maiden on the voyage." Henry pitched his voice deeper and held his nose up in the air. "If any man on the ship shows interest in my Idee, I shall give him a thorough appraisal."

Their carriage passed through New York's busy streets toward the port. Ida chuckled at Henry's dramatics. "I hardly can think of a suitor or my future at the moment," Ida said. "I need to take care of Marmee, not think about myself."

Henry raised his eyebrows, pointed to his mouth full of peanuts, and shrugged.

Ida blew the hair falling on her forehead. Would this trip turn her into an old maid? "I will be stuck in India during my best courting years."

"Nonsense." Henry swallowed and shook his head. "You never know what God has in mind for you."

The carriage stopped outside the Port of New York. Henry paid the driver and helped him unload the trunks.

Ida and Henry joined the line of passengers waiting at the ticket office. Ida reached into her purse and unfolded the pre-purchased ticket.

City of Berlin
July 30, 1890
Destination: Liverpool, England

A throng of people lined up at multiple ticket windows. The room was a hive of voices. People pressed from behind as they moved forward a step at a time for their turn.

Ida pulled at Henry's sleeve. "Do you think I should stay in New York, find a hospital for Marmee, and you bring her back?"

Tilting his head, Henry's smile disappeared. "I don't understand."

"We're still in New York. I could forfeit my ticket." Ida pursed her lips. "A church could help me until you and Marmee returned."

"Wait for us? That's at least four or five months." He took her hand and held her attention with his eyes. "You're nervous, sis. That's all."

Ida and her brother were next in line to board. Ida rested a finger against her lips for a moment. She didn't want to tell Henry how much she deplored India. "I don't want to feel obligated. I wish I wanted to go." Ida huffed and slumped her shoulders. "Never mind. I'm rambling."

Ida watched the ticket master stamp Henry's ticket. She took a deep breath and passed her ticket through the window. She'd nearly worn a hole in the paper from holding it so tight.

The man stamped Ida's ticket. "You'll change ships in Liverpool," the ticket master said. "Your trunks are automatically transferred for you."

Ida and Henry scooted to the side and walked toward the door leading to the dock. Outside, seagulls dived at the water. The waves sloshed against the pier's columns. Barnacles looked like rocks stuck against the heavy timber. Henry stopped and gently steered Ida's shoulders to face him. "Apprehension is natural. Moving to India is a big change for both of us."

"This move isn't permanent for me, so I need assurance. Am I doing the right thing? I've prayed, hoping God will show me that I've made the right decision." Ida looked out toward the ocean. "And more than anything else, I've prayed for Marmee."

Henry patted the top of Ida's hand. "You've made the best decision. I've worried I won't be a suitable teacher for the boys' school in India." Henry sounded gentle and kind. "Our parents, our mentors, and our prayers guide us."

"You mean I'm doing the right thing even if I'm not completely enthusiastic?"

"Exactly. We can't base hard decisions on feelings. The Bible cautions us not to rely on our hearts. God is our guide."

"Yes, God is in control." Ida lifted her chin. "Shall we go?"

After a short walk, she and Henry joined the line in front of the gangplank. Ida studied the black hulk of the steamship while they waited to board. The wide-open spaces of the Northfield hillsides were gone. The throng of people waiting to board reminded her of ants hovering over a spilled crumb. Her heart pounded.

"If I were a princess, I'd abdicate my duty. Hold my hand tight," she said to Henry. "I still want to run."

CHAPTER 4

Within an hour, Ida and Henry stood on the ship's deck along with hundreds of passengers and waved to the crowd on the dock. Ocean spray misted the passengers. When the ship moved into the Atlantic, the water changed color from gray to deep blue.

Henry wrapped an arm around Ida's shoulders. "Won't it be good to be back to our birthplace? We're going home, Idee."

"America is my home, not India. All I remember of India is . . ." Her voice dropped. "Dying children." How could her brother have such a different view of the same place? "I can't grasp how you feel the least bit fond of India."

Henry leaned on the ship's railing.

"I plan to bring Marmee back to the States with me," Ida said, "after my four years of service is completed."

Henry unbuttoned his vest and checked his pocket watch. "Time for supper." He placed Ida's hand over his forearm and led her to the dining room. When they arrived, he pulled the chair out for Ida to sit. He took the seat to her left. A candle flickered in the middle of the formal dining table.

A server hovered beside Ida and set rolls on the bread plates and a pot of tea in the middle of the table. Henry took her hand. "Let's trust God with Marmee's welfare and your future. I'll bless our food." He bowed his head and prayed.

The candle cast spots of light against the glasses. Ida stared at the light. Trust? She felt her emotions rising like the waves. *How can I trust God when, so far, nothing in my life has gone the way I intended?*

Ida placed a pat of butter on the roll and spread it over the bread.

"Slow down there, Idee. You've made a hole in the bread." Henry chuckled.

"Where was my family when my time to step out into society as a debutante arrived?" She waved her hands in the air.

The server served Ida and Henry a warm plate of chicken, mashed potatoes, and lima beans. Henry smothered his potatoes with gravy. "Idee, our family isn't high society."

Ida's words tumbled out like a waterfall. Years of resentment against her parents for leaving her to attend school floated to the tip of her tongue. "Now, when I've finally grown comfortable living away from family—why have I been pulled back? If Father and Marmee want to be missionaries, so be it. Under the circumstances, I am happy to serve, but I will not be the next Scudder to carry on the family legacy of missionaries."

Henry chewed the chicken like he hadn't eaten in years.

Ida poked at the lima beans with her fork. "What if Marmee dies?" There. She'd said the words she'd kept locked up in her mind.

Henry set his fork down and held Ida's hand. "I've worried too, but," his voice took on a tender tone, "prayer is our only resource."

Ida searched her brother's face from his red crew cut and blue eyes to the whiskers on his chin. "You remind me of Father's sunny attitude."

Less than two weeks later, the ship disembarked in Liverpool, England. From there Ida and Henry transferred to a ship bound for India.

Ida stayed on deck to watch while it traveled through the Strait of Gibraltar. After Gibraltar, the ship entered the Mediterranean Sea until it reached Port Said six days later at the opening of the Suez Canal.

A week later they made it through the Red Sea. Before moving into the deep waters of the Arabian Sea, the ship dropped anchor at the red cliffs of the Aden peninsula to replenish coal for the steam engine.

Ida and Henry stood on the deck to watch while the ship bunkered. The vibration of the giant propellers, the throbbing engines, and the smell of the smokestacks stopped when the ship berthed. Ida heard voices from the shore but couldn't understand their language.

"Look, camels are carrying the coal in baskets on their backs." Henry pointed to the shore.

The camels crouched on the sand. Men loaded the coal baskets from the camels onto a barge. Loaded with coal, the barge floated out to the ship with the men. The men passed the baskets to the ship crew, who poured the coal into chutes.

If Ida wasn't sightseeing from the deck, she spent her days reading, writing in her journal, and joining games of checkers or shuffleboard. After breakfast each morning, Ida and Henry met on the deck for Bible study.

A few people sitting nearby asked to join. Before long, about a dozen passengers gathered on the deck for morning worship with Henry and Ida.

On September 20, the ship ported in Madras, India. A guide dismissed one section at a time on the ship. Ida and Henry waited among hundreds to exit. They watched from the deck while others reunited with their loved ones. Ida slid her hands into her white gloves and adjusted her hat. *God, will you show me how to trust you?*

Voices filled the air with people hailing porters to gather their trunks or catch a ride on a bullock cart. Ida gulped. Her throat tightened. She was in India. Within a few minutes, she'd see her father for the first time in eight long years.

Henry's eyes lit up. "Our section is next."

Half her life she'd vowed never to come back to India. A jumble of excitement and dread, she didn't know how to respond to Henry's eagerness. How could he be so happy, when she was so doubtful?

She watched the passengers ahead of them make their way down the gangplank toward a throng waiting on the platform. Where was Father?

"At last, we're moving," Henry said, taking Ida's hand and escorting her down the gangplank.

When they reached the deck, Ida steadied herself and searched the crowd. Women with long braids and silken saris, holding babies on their backs, glided past. Vendors sold brass and silver trinkets. Women squatted around bowls of chili peppers, cardamom pods, and dried pepper berries. Their heads were covered with bright fuchsia, sunshine yellow, and sea blue saris.

Most men walked barefoot and wore long white tunics with pants underneath. Other men wore only a white loin cloth and a turban. Errand boys zigzagged past swarms of people. Men with large loads on their backs trotted through the streets.

Each sight and smell reminded Ida of her childhood. "Where's Father?"

A line of sweat trickled down Henry's face. "He may be the only person with a Western suit on."

"Plus his unmistakable beard and round spectacles." Ida pulled off her gloves and fanned the hot air around her face.

"There!" Henry pointed and pulled Ida in the direction of a strange man.

A stooped-shouldered man walked toward them. He looked shorter than her father. And his wrinkled face looked too old.

"Come on, Idee." Henry tugged at her hand.

Ida planted her feet in the ground like a stubborn horse. "That man is not my father."

CHAPTER 5

Ida bounded past the stranger.

"My beautiful girl."

The voice belonged to her daddy. Ida stopped in mid-step and turned in the direction of the voice.

"My dear, it's me." The stranger's brown eyes looked identical to Father's, but who was this frail man with a long white beard?

She took a step toward him. "Father?" Ida's voice cracked.

"Yes." He tugged at his beard, reached for Ida, and wrapped her in his arms.

A mix of emotions confused her. She wanted to cry on her father's shoulder and tell him how good it was to be with him. At the same time, she wanted to look right in his eyes—for now she was as tall as he—and scold him for leaving her. Could she forgive him?

Father gently released her and stepped back. He tugged on a handkerchief in his front pocket, lifted his glasses, and wiped his eyes. "Two of my children right beside me again."

Henry clapped Father's back and wrapped him in a hug.

Tears stung Ida's eyes. That man with the quivering chin was Father. No matter how many years she'd spent away from him, seeing him face to face reminded her how dearly she loved him. She grabbed his hand and pressed it tight.

"We're eighty miles from Tindivanam. I'll hire a *jutka* to take us to the Madras train station." Father spoke to one of the drivers clustered around several carriages harnessed to horses. Ida and Henry climbed into a lemon-yellow jutka with orange marigolds decorating the sides. Another jutka carried their trunks. The drivers climbed onto a seat in front of the carriage and directed the bullocks forward.

Within fifteen minutes, the three arrived at the Madras train station and boarded a train for Tindivanam. Ida's heart chugged like the tempo of the train. Rust-colored dust blew through the open car. Palm trees clustered around thatched-roof villages. "Why didn't I remember how pretty the rice fields are? They shine like emeralds."

"Everything looked brown from famine when we left, dear. But you've arrived in monsoon season. We've had plenty of rain to green up the fields."

Ida's stomach clenched. Marmee's poor health weighed heavy on her mind. She shut her eyes and prayed to herself. *Dear Lord, keep Marmee alive.*

Almost three hours later, the train rounded past a thick tamarind forest. "I spot the depot." Henry nudged Ida with his elbow.

Ida's heart pounded. "Are we close to the mission?"

"The mission is about thirty minutes from town," Father said.

Five years since she'd seen Marmee. Thirty more minutes wasn't so long to wait. A lump formed in Ida's throat.

The train screeched to a stop. Ida stepped out ahead of Henry and her father. Ida tugged at her high-necked collar. She fanned herself, but the air felt hotter than the furnace that heated Northfield dormitory for winter.

"Idee, you should see yourself. Your hair's covered with dust from the roads. You're a brownish redhead now." Henry flashed Ida a teasing grin. "But, no amount of dirt could cover your beauty, sister." He wiped a smudge of dirt off her nose.

Sweat stains had turned her dress from satin blue to violet gray. Her muttonchop sleeves had deflated and stuck to her arms. Ida swiped at her hair to shake the dust away.

"Our last ride." Father pointed to the oxcarts lined alongside the dirt road where drivers stood waiting for business.

Each bandy wagon had a reed canopy and was harnessed to a bullock. Ida climbed into the bandy wagon. Father and Henry squeezed in next to Ida.

"*Hinh. Hinh.*" The driver prodded the bullock. But no amount of wishing, calling, or prodding changed the bullock's speed.

Ida swallowed. Fear of the unknown knotted at her stomach. She kept her eyes focused on the palm tree fronds, pink oleanders, and the vining bougainvilleas.

The procession passed through a narrow gate, the wheels crunching over the dirt road. In the distance Ida spotted a small white building with a thatched roof. Was the silhouette on the porch Marmee?

Ida refused to wait another second. The bandy wagon moved too slow. "Marmee!" She slid out of

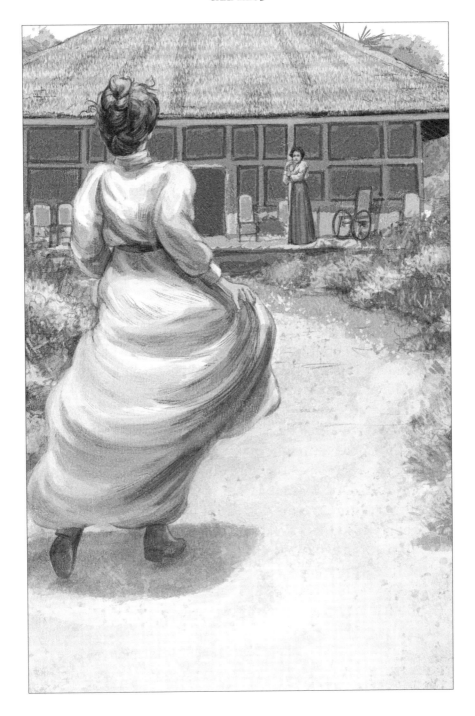

the moving wagon and ran past the tamarind trees toward the porch.

Marmee held the porch column. Her dark hair parted in the middle and the silver brooch was pinned to her dress, as always.

The words Ida longed to say in person tumbled out. She wrapped her arms around her mother. "At last, I'm with you."

The sweet scent of her mother washed over her. Shivers ran up her arms. Ida kept her head buried in her mother's shoulder for a couple of minutes until she raised her head and wiped the tears from her eyes.

Like she did when Ida was a little girl, Marmee rubbed Ida's back. "I knew I'd live to see you again."

Ida's insides pinched.

"I worked as long as I could," Marmee's voice wavered, "but your father put me to bed. I asked him to send for you." She stopped to catch her breath.

Ida grabbed Marmee's arm. "You need to rest."

Marmee pointed to the far end of the veranda. Three doors faced the drive. "The door closest to us is your room. The middle door opens to the main house, and my bedroom is the third door down."

Ida clasped her mother's arm. Could she even walk the three yards to the door? Nothing could have prepared her for how sick Marmee was. Ida's eyes stung. She batted the tears back. At least, she reminded herself, Marmee was alive.

When they reached the bedroom, Ida eased her mother into bed and leaned her against a pillow.

"Are you comfortable?" Ida swallowed hard. Emotionally, reversing roles wasn't as easy as she'd expected.

"Yes, thank you, dearest."

Ida touched the whitewashed walls and looked up at the thatched ceiling. Compared to the bungalow where they'd lived when she was little, this one looked more primitive.

"I'm so relieved you're here." Marmee blew out a long, rattled breath. "I worried your father might work himself to death. He needs help. He's kept up with all of my jobs, his patients, and his preaching." She paused and sucked in a breath. "We closed the schools temporarily."

Ida knew Father was a hard worker. He'd always risen early. Always overworked. But through his glasses, Ida noticed the bags under his eyes. A pang of guilt pricked at her for wishing she didn't have to come. How could she have been so selfish?

"And I worried about you and Henry traveling so far." Marmee sighed. "But here you are in the flesh. An answered prayer."

Ida wiped her eyes with the back of her hand. "Yes, I'm here." She rubbed Marmee's hand. "I'm going to find Henry."

Ida found Father and Henry unloading a trunk beside a door at the other end of the veranda. Ida waved Henry in her direction. "Marmee's in here."

Henry ran and, when he reached her, Ida took his hand and led him inside the bedroom with Father close behind.

Marmee put her hands to her cheeks. "My son." Tears flooded her face.

Ida and Father smiled at each other while Henry embraced Marmee.

The four talked for over an hour. Father led the conversation with important news. "Did you notice the construction across the street?" Father said. "We're going to live in a two-storied *pukka*."

25

Ida scrunched her face. "Pukka?"

"A real house, not thatched," Henry said. "I still recognize some of the Tamil." He stood and motioned for Ida to take his place beside Marmee.

"I wish I remembered," Ida said. She dreaded taking language lessons. How long before she'd understand anyone?

"The mission house will have a tiled roof and concrete walls," Father said, smiling.

Ida noticed Marmee's face looked chalky white like the whitewashed walls in the bungalow. She placed her hands on Marmee's cheeks. "Your skin is cold."

"Will you pull the blanket tight around my shoulders?" Marmee said, shivering.

"The effects of malaria," Father said. "Daily chills, headaches, sweats, and weakness. She's past the fever, but the symptoms last four to six months, sometimes up to nine." Father and Ida helped Marmee scoot beneath the covers. "Let's give her time to rest."

"Absolutely." Henry blew a kiss to Marmee.

"Ida?"

"Yes?"

"You were just a girl when I left you with Uncle Henry. You're a young woman now." Marmee whispered. "I'd never—"

Ida took her mother's hands in hers. "I'm so happy to be with you again. Nothing else matters."

"We couldn't offer you a proper education in India. We didn't want you in India for fear of another famine. At the time it made sense to leave you with family." Marmee shook her head. "Your father and I agreed we'd never leave you again. I'm sorry."

"Please, don't wear yourself out," Ida said.

Ida stroked her mother's back, thankful Father had summoned her to help. "I love you." The awareness of her mother's sacrifice seemed so obvious. Why hadn't it occurred to her before? "You had to make hard decisions," she whispered.

Marmee had fallen asleep, her chest rattling with each breath. Ida kissed Marmee's cheek, rose from the edge of the bed, and tiptoed out.

Father led Henry and Ida outside and stopped. He turned and took Ida's hand. A fresh batch of tears seeped from behind Father's wireframe glasses. "I agree with your mother's sentiments. I hope you'll forgive me for leaving you behind, especially for asking your mother to join me."

She wasn't prepared to forgive Father, but looking in his face made the bitterness she'd harbored loosen its grip. How could she stay angry? Ida gently squeezed his hand. "Of course, Father, I forgive you."

He led them to the middle door on the veranda and opened it. "We use this room for an office. I study for sermons, review medical journals, and entertain visitors."

Ida sniffed. "Something smells like popcorn." Ida walked toward the back of the room to an open door.

Behind the office, a woman squatted beside a mound of stones on the ground with fire in the middle. A pot simmered over the fire. "This covered area is our kitchen. The mission employs several workers, including cooks. We serve meals to both the boys' and girls' school every day."

Father walked them outside to the back of the mission house. "Henry and Ida, I'd like you to meet, Salomi Benjamin." Ida and Henry smiled while Father repeated the introduction in Tamil.

"Salomi and her father are both Christians and work for the mission. Salomi speaks some English, so she may communicate with you on a limited basis."

"What's cooking?" Ida squatted next to Salomi.

"*Arici.*" Salomi lifted the lid.

"Rice. I remember the smell, and, finally, I recognize a word."

A few minutes later, Father, Henry, and Ida enjoyed the curry and rice in the office. Ida took a deep breath, trying to stay alert.

"You've both had a long day," Father said. "I see your eyes blinking, Ida."

She took a deep breath. "I don't usually like to retire before dark, but all I want is to clean off this grime and sleep."

"In the morning, I'll walk you both through the daily chores. Henry, your accommodations are here." Father pointed to a cushion on the floor and stood. "Follow me, dear, and I'll show you the bedroom."

Ida and Father walked back to the veranda. Outside, the birds tweeted their evening songs, flying back and forth among the tamarind trees. Father opened the door at the far end. A double, metal-framed bed, a desk, and bedside table with an oil lamp furnished the room.

"An *almirah* for your clothes." Father opened the double doors on the freestanding closet. He walked to the corner, opened a door, and stepped to the side for Ida to see. "And a bathing area."

Ida peered into a small cement shower stall with a hole in the middle.

"That's an open drain." Father shut the door. "Always check the drain for spiders or a snake before you take a shower."

Ida's gasped. "And what do I do if there's a—a— living thing in my shower stall?" Her heart thumped. Another good reason to detest India.

"Back away and call for help." Father chuckled. "I'm sure you'll not run into any harm."

"Thank you for bringing me back to Marmee."

Father embraced Ida.

Ida held Father a little longer. "I can't believe it's really you." Tears pooled in her eyes. She sniffed and let her arms drop.

Father kissed her on the forehead. "Sleep well, sweet one." He turned and closed the door.

She swallowed the lump in her throat. Too weary to read or write letters, Ida searched her trunk pushed against the wall beside her bed until she found a fresh nightgown. She sniffed the clean cotton scent and the lavender sachets she'd stored in the trunk. After she washed her face in the basin, she decided to cut short her nightly routine of combing her hair a hundred strokes.

Every muscle in her body relaxed when she climbed beneath the sheet. She stared at the ceiling while she thought over the day. A brown lizard, the size of her hand, scurried across the thatch and down the wall and up again. Then down again. Yes, she was definitely in India. A clump of dirt spiraled down and smacked her in the forehead. She shot out of bed, back to the basin, and cleaned her face again.

She stomped to the bed. Had she traveled thousands of miles to endure dirt falling on her bed and listen to lizards as bedtime companions? Here she was in India, where she couldn't speak the language. And where she'd vowed to never live again.

CHAPTER 6

Ida woke to a light tap on the door. She yawned, rubbed her eyes, and sat up. Nothing seemed familiar. Where was Florence? Annie? She looked around the dark room. Her eyes focused on the trunk, reminding her she wasn't in Northfield anymore. Another tap. Ida pulled herself out of bed, shrugged into her robe, and opened the door a crack.

"*Chota. Ammal.*" Salomi held a steaming cup of coffee, banana, and a plate of bread.

Ida swung the door open wide.

Salomi stepped inside, set the chota on the desk, and lit the lantern. "Dr. John said to wake you, Ammal."

"Thank you for the coffee."

Salomi put both hands together, bowed, and shut the door.

Ida opened her trunk and quickly slipped into an outfit. She chose a brown skirt and white shirt. Balancing the breakfast and lantern in her hands, she hurried to the office. A light rain had wet the outer edge of the porch.

Father stood at his desk and poured medicine from a large brown jug into a smaller bottle. "Good morning, my darling." He turned to a glass cabinet on the side wall, returned the medicine bottle, and retrieved another. "I hope you slept well."

"In spite of a lizard, I slept as content as a kitten." Ida set the plate and lantern on a table. She sipped the coffee. "Is Marmee awake?"

Father glanced at the clock. "Afraid not, dear. She didn't sleep well. I told her to stay in bed until you woke her." He held the brown glass jug over the funnel, while the last dribbles dropped into the bottle. "I'll need to telegraph the mission in Madras for more supplies when I go to town. I'm low on ether, quinine, and chloroform."

She studied Father. Even with the Santa Claus features she'd always loved, his suit hung looser around his stomach. From her childhood memories, Father was a devoted doctor. Why did he choose India to practice medicine? No matter. She loved him dearly, even if she didn't always understand his choices.

A stack of white cloths lay in a basket on the desk. She scooped a cloth and folded it into a rectangle. "Let me help fold the bandages. I remember Marmee boiled the bandages every day when we lived in Nebraska."

"Marmee is an excellent assistant."

Henry turned over on his floor pallet. "How can the two of you sound so chipper this early?"

"It's daybreak. Nearly time to work." Father chuckled. "Where's your rise and shine? The day's getting away. Salomi delivered your coffee already."

Ida handed Henry his coffee. "It's getting cold."

Henry chugged a swallow. "Ugh." He scowled. "Maybe I'll go beg for a fresh cup."

The smell of bread cakes cooking outside wafted through the window. Henry walked to the back kitchen area, returned with a steaming cup, and sat on a chair.

Finished folding, Ida took a seat beside Henry and nibbled her bread.

"Let's discuss the jobs that need immediate attention." Father gave a sheet of paper to Henry and Ida. "I've referenced most of the chores here."

Henry whistled. "Impressive list."

"Once I knew you were coming, I logged the jobs. The how-to details you can hear from Marmee. Henry, your first duty is the laundry at the boys' school. You will gather the dirty clothes, bag, and deliver them to the *dhobi*."

"Dhobi?" Henry said.

"Washerwoman."

Father looked at Ida. "The school is here on the mission compound. I'm going to take Henry over to introduce him. I'll send him back before the noon meal. Will you check on Marmee first?"

She smiled. "I'm happy to take care of Marmee."

"We feed a hundred boys every day at the school. At lunch," he looked at Henry, "you and Ida will deliver the meals to the boys."

Father unlocked a desk drawer and opened a box with coins and a few bills. "Ida, the money is here. My driver, Souri, will take you to the bazaar to shop later this morning."

When she heard a noise outside, Ida leaned to look out the window.

Henry walked to the window. "We have a visitor."

A horse-drawn wagon stopped in front of the bungalow. An Indian man hopped off the wagon seat and held the ponies' reins.

"My driver." Father grabbed his doctor bag and walked outside with Ida and Henry in tow where Father made introductions.

The morning sun glistened against the wet leaves on the trees. A dog barked in the distance. Memories of living in India as a seven-year-old girl weren't the same as what she was seeing. The trees and plants were lusher. She remembered brown. Dead trees. Dead animals. And dead people.

Ida took a deep breath and cupped her hand around her ear. "I hear voices."

"Ah, Tindivanam is coming alive." Father paused. "People are headed into town for work, which I must do as well." Father beamed at Ida and Henry. "It's so wonderful to have my children at home."

Ida smiled.

After Souri and Father left, Ida's heart jumped. Time to see Marmee.

———

Ida tried not to spill the coffee as she walked to her parents' bedroom. She tapped on the door, then opened it.

Flared against the pillow, Marmee's hair looked like hay scattered on a barn floor. Ida stifled a gasp. She'd rarely seen her mother's hair down. Her white night dress matched the shade of her skin tone. "Time to wake," Ida whispered.

"My dream is here." Marmee smiled. "Come here."

Even though fright hummed through her, Ida did her best to grin. What if Marmee died? Seeing her mother, a lioness of a woman, tucked in the shelter of a bed made her want to melt into a puddle of tears. Ida helped her up. "Ready for breakfast?"

"I'm not hungry."

Ida rubbed her hand across Marmee's forehead. "You have a fever."

"Don't be alarmed." Marmee took a haggard breath. "Fever is my companion." She paused. "My medicine. On the bureau." Another breath. "It helps."

Ida moved off the bed, found directions on a note, and spooned a dose of quinine from the bottle. Holding her hand underneath the spoon, she placed the liquid to Marmee's lips. Then she took a washrag, dipped it in a bowl of water, and laid it across her mother's forehead.

"Will you make sure to distribute . . ." She paused. "Sixty measures of rice." Marmee's voice sounded weaker.

"Sh-sh-sh. I can ask Salomi how." Ida poured water from the jar in the room. "Here, take a sip." She held the cup to Marmee's mouth.

She put her head back. "I want to explain the jobs, but—"

"Rest, please." Ida set the glass of water on the bureau and smoothed Marmee's hair off her face.

"Check supplies. Shop."

"Don't worry." Ida massaged her mother's temples. "Father wrote out the chores." She couldn't tell mother that she didn't know how to do the chores. She'd figure it out. "You're going to get better," Ida whispered. *Dear God, please let my words be true.*

Marmee closed her eyes and fell asleep. Ida knelt beside the bed and prayed. *I'm here, God. Please don't take my mother now.* Her throat tightened. Seeing

Marmee so weak and tired alarmed her. Was she strong enough to care for her sick mother?

After praying for several minutes, Ida stood. When she got to the door, she turned back. "If there's anything in my power—no, in God's power—you will be the lioness of the Scudder family once again."

CHAPTER 7

She climbed into the wagon with Souri and held a list of supplies for the mission. Ida wished for the first time she knew how to speak Tamil. Shopping at the market would not be easy. But duty called.

"I don't know the language or the money system," she said. "Are you ready for an adventure?"

"I will help you, Ammal," Souri said.

Fifteen minutes later Souri parked the wagon near the end of a busy dirt street. Down the bazaar, vendors sat on the mats beside their fruits and vegetables, a sea of greens, yellows, oranges, and reds. Nearby, a cow tied to a tree branch rested in the shade. Flower petals covered the ground around the cow. At the corner of the crowded street, twenty yards away, a woman crouched.

"What is she doing?" Ida said.

"She is sprinkling ash on the cow dung."

With a flat piece of tin, she scraped the pile into a basket, and then swept the area clean with a hand broom. The sweeper continued past them and avoided eye contact.

"She's barefoot, and the street's so dirty." Ida wanted to wash the lady's feet and buy her a pair of sandals. "I know cows are sacred to the Hindu, but she shouldn't have to clea—" Ida exploded out of the wagon and strode toward the sweeper.

"Please wait, Ammal." Souri followed her and held his arm out. "You cannot stop her. She is a street sweeper."

Ida held her lips tight, closed her eyes tight, and blew out a breath. Down the bazaar, other women sold merchandise and produce at their street stands. No one noticed the sweeper.

"The Hindu's believe she is an untouchable. From birth, she's taught to do this work," Souri said.

Ida sighed. Why, oh, why did a person have to earn a wage by sweeping after cows? She and Souri entered the busy bazaar.

Loud and shrill, vendors called to shoppers. Babies squalled, wrapped inside their mothers' saris. Bells clanged from the temple towering against the sky. Vendors sat cross-legged beside mounds of mangoes, bananas, grapes, and guava, all neatly displayed on mats.

Ida stopped and squeezed a mango to check the ripeness.

"*Māṅkani.* Mangoes," Souri said.

She selected mangoes and bananas, repeating each word as Souri identified them in Tamil. Ida opened her change purse, and Souri counted the coins for her. While Souri talked with the vendor, Ida concentrated on the conversation to learn a few Tamil words.

The next vendor sat under a lean-to roof made of reed, suspended on bamboo stalks. Ida browsed through the displays of brass bells, Buddha statues, and silver jewelry.

Dogs and goats walked among the people. When a cow meandered through the street, the crowd pressed closer to the shops to widen the path.

An Indian woman in her long silk sari held a silver bangle and slid it on Ida's wrist. She ran her hand over Ida's arm and smiled, her front teeth missing.

"No, thank you." Ida smiled, shook her head, and slid the bracelet off. She wanted to buy the bracelet but didn't have spending money.

The woman held a necklace in the air, flaunting it in front of Ida's face. "Pretty."

"*Paravāyillai, naṉṟi*. No, thank you," Souri said and motioned for Ida.

"Why can't the street sweeper work in the market like these other women?" Ida couldn't get her mind off the street sweeper. She'd never dream of spending her life sweeping after cows. "Didn't that woman know how many other jobs she could choose?"

"People live by the tradition," Souri said. "She is a sweeper because of her birth."

"I know about the caste system." Ida stopped at the next vendor and sniffed fresh cinnamon drying in the sun. "But a lady shouldn't be allowed to do such work. It's dishonorable."

"Before Dr. John told me the story of Jesus' sacrifice, I swept the streets." Souri beamed and patted his heart. "Now I am Christian. I am free because of my new birth. I am a son of Jesus. The mission gives me work, so I do not sweep anymore."

Ida leaned over bowls of cloves, turmeric, ginger, vanilla pods, and curry leaves, thinking about everything she'd seen. Something inside her wanted to help the poor woman.

Ida and Souri moved on and stopped at a vendor where flowers draped over wood panels gave off a wonderful fragrance. She sniffed. "I adore the scent of gardenias." She ran her hand gently across the garland. "I've seen the delightful and the dreadful all in one day."

Ida opened her change purse, selected a garland, and watched Souri show her the correct coins to pay. She laid the flowers in her basket on top of the fruits like she had a baby in her hands. "I know someone who loves flowers as much as I do."

Shopping completed, Ida and Souri walked back to the wagon and returned to the mission. When they arrived home, Ida checked on Marmee, helped her dress, and walked her to the veranda to eat lunch.

Ida wrapped the garland around Marmee's neck. "For the queen."

"What lovely flowers." Marmee kissed Ida's cheek. "How kind. I'm hardly a queen, but you are a princess. The sight of you is more beautiful than any flower God made."

Ida grinned at Marmee and sat in the rocker next to her. "You're always a queen to me." After resting for a few minutes, Ida rose. "I'll be back as soon as I help Henry deliver the meals to the boys' school."

An hour later, Ida joined Marmee on the veranda for lunch. Across the street, men and woman sat under trees, eating, sleeping, or talking. Near a clump of cactuses, a green dove cooed and pecked at the ground, looking for seeds.

"Is it time for afternoon chores?" Ida said.

"The sun says it's time. Will you check the *godown*?" Marmee explained the steps to clean the rice storage shed. "We want to keep pests out. The weevils aren't hard to catch, but you'll have to take a lantern with you to see the grubs."

"Grubs?"

"Tiny white larvae. They look like rice except they wiggle and have a brown head. Checking the godown isn't a job for a weak stomach." She patted Ida's arm, and smoothed out the wrinkles in her long, black skirt. "I'd like to sit with Salomi in the kitchen. At least I can chop vegetables for dinner."

Ida dreaded picking bugs out of rice bags but didn't let her voice reveal her angst. "I'm not sure I'll do the work as well as you, but I'm not afraid." She eased Marmee out of the rocker and followed the path to the back. "Am I walking too fast?"

Marmee shook her head. "The pace is too slow for my liking, but my body won't move any faster."

They rounded the corner of the bungalow. "I didn't realize there were so many more buildings here," Ida said.

"The other mission buildings house the workers, the animals, and store our grain," Marmee said. She paused to catch her breath. "We have four Indian families, all Christians, working here. Your Father built each building." Another pause. "He wants to give every new Christian a job and a bungalow."

When they reached the cooking hut, Ida helped settle Marmee on the floor mat and handed her a knife and a bowl of okra to chop alongside Salomi and Mrs. Benjamin. Ida grabbed the brass water vessel and a few minutes later, covered her hair with a scarf, slid on a pair of gloves, and climbed up the short ladder into the thatched-roof godown. The late afternoon sun shone through the open-air windows at the top.

Burlap rice bags were stacked on top of a wood platform. Ida spotted a weevil, about the size of a fly, hovering over a bag. She caught it with her fingers and dropped it in the water. Why was she chosen to pick bugs off rice bags? This work wasn't any less disgusting than the street sweeper's.

The verse in Colossians 3 came to mind: "Whatsoever ye do, do it heartily, as to the Lord, and not unto men."

She snatched another weevil and dropped it in the water. *I am doing this work for you, Lord, but I'm not happy about it.* Ida stood in this stifling prison of burlap while her friends probably wore new dresses and stood arm-in-arm next to boyfriends, dining on lobster bisque. Beads of sweat formed a necklace around her throat. Ida vowed she would never live like this and forfeit a comfortable life in America.

An hour later her white gloves were stained brown, her apron plastered with squished grubs, and the water vessel black from the drowned weevils. One step at a time, she wobbled down the ladder, trying not to spill the bug water on her dress. Her legs ached from squatting to inspect the rice bags.

When she reached the veranda, she jerked off the filthy gloves and apron, and threw them in a pile at her feet. Why had she worn her good gloves?

In her room, the mirror reflected her dirty face. Tears crept over her cheeks, painting smudged rivers on her face. What happened to her porcelain skin? She stomped to the bed and crumpled in a heap. She was mad for missing all the fun back home, but she wanted to help Marmee. How could one day of duty already make her want to quit? Her fists pounded the bed. *Why God? I'm not the person for this job. How long will I have to stay in this dreadful place?*

On Sunday several people had already gathered near the door of the church when Father and Ida arrived.

"I built the church myself when I first came back." Father smiled and stood tall, rubbing a hand over the brick wall of the building that stood not far from their bungalow on the mission property.

"Real brick and tile. I remember you fixing the barn in Nebraska. You can do anything, can't you, Father?"

"Working with my hands gives me great satisfaction, but not as much as ministering to people. Let's go inside."

Father led Ida inside the church. The waiting people followed them. Ida watched the congregation gather on mats covering the dirt floor and recognized several who worked at the mission.

A lady who smelled liked coconut hung a garland around Ida's shoulders. "*Mikka makilcci*, so happy," the lady said.

Father grinned. "Last week during church, I told the parishioners to expect you here this week."

"*Dorai sani*? Mrs. John," another visitor said.

"*Illai*. No. I insisted she rest this morning," Father said.

Ida watched the crowd coming, hoping she'd see the street sweeper from the bazaar. Families of five or six and a smattering of a few singles slowly filled the room. A few minutes before the service started, Henry arrived with the boys from the school. Ida estimated the room held several hundred people, but she didn't recognize anyone except people who worked at the mission. "Are they all Christians?"

"No, we only have four Christian families, but I'm happy to see all the visitors. I'll begin the service with hymns," Father said.

"Am I expected to play? My musical skills aren't noteworthy." She laughed. "Sometimes I don't hit all the right notes."

Father winked and walked to the front of the room behind his podium.

Ida climbed on the bench, pumping the pedal several times on the portable organ. She'd be thrilled to see Marmee well enough to take over the music. Ida wiped her hands on her skirt and played. She cringed at her efforts to keep time with her father. She hit the wrong key a few times, as she expected, but no one seemed to notice her nervous hands.

When Father led the congregation in "Blessed Assurance," Ida sang in English while she played. She didn't have assurance of anything. Would Marmee live? Would she ever get to leave India?

They reached the second stanza. She sang, but the words stung. "Perfect submission, all is at rest." Her soul wasn't at rest. Her mind wouldn't submit. Her body might be in India, but her heart wasn't.

God must know she was a hypocrite.

CHAPTER 8

1891
One Year Later

One October evening, Ida joined Marmee in the office while Father was in town visiting patients. Ida sat beside Marmee, admiring her meticulous stitching. The lines straight and taut, Marmee hemmed a baby gown.

"Shall I read in Psalms where we stopped last night?" Ida said.

Marmee smiled and focused on the task at hand. "Please do."

"We're on Psalm sixteen." Ida flipped the pages of her Bible open and began to read. "'Therefore my heart is glad, and my glory rejoiceth.'" When she reached verse nine she stopped to write a note in her journal.

Marmee's face glowed in the lamp light.

"My heart is glad tonight. Your cheeks have a rosy tint instead of blanched white. I rejoice each day you get better."

"I believe in miracles," Marmee said.

"Watching you recover has strengthened my relationship with the Lord. You're an answer to prayer. When I first got here, you could hardly breathe. Now look at you."

"I'm gaining strength each day."

Ida smoothed her hand over the Bible then continued reading verses ten and eleven. "'Thou wilt show me the path of life.'" She stopped and underlined verse eleven. "Do you believe God will show me my path?"

Marmee set the gown on her lap and leaned forward. "Open your heart to God's plan."

"I don't know what I want to do with my life." She shrugged. "I have three more years here with you in India before I need to know what my future holds."

"If you pray for His guidance, God will lead you." Marmee snipped the white thread, set the needle in the pin cushion, and tied a knot. "I sew as many of these baptismal gowns as I can before Father takes a trip to the villages." She pressed the folds of the fabric down in her lap. "I dress the infants when they're baptized."

Ida lifted the gown. "It's so tiny."

"The babies are so beautiful. A headful of dark hair and big brown eyes. Ah, if only I could travel on the next trip." Marmee leaned her head back and smiled.

Ida looked at the contentment on Marmee's face. She'd seen that look before when Marmee helped people who came to the mission. Ida cupped her hand around her ear. "Sounds like a soft rain outside."

"I hope your Father makes it home before the rain gets heavy."

Ida walked to the window. "I see a light down the road. Must be the lantern wobbling on the wagon."

Marmee found another unfinished gown in the sewing box, threaded a needle, and began hemming. "I think you ought to help Father on his next trip in November. He's traveling after monsoon season ends."

"I couldn't leave you." Ida set the gown on the table and returned to her chair.

"Henry is next door at the school. Souri, Salomi, and everyone else here will help. If you go, you'll be with Uncle Jared and Dixie."

"I would truly love to see my favorite cousin."

Marmee smiled, pulling the thread in and out of the white cloth.

The door opened. Father took off his hat, swiped it with his handkerchief, and hung it on the clothes tree. Drops of rain dripped from his hat to the floor.

"Glad you are home, dear," Marmee said. "How did your visit go?"

Father slumped into a chair and sighed. "Sad case. A woman with severe eye pain."

"Did they let you examine her?" Ida said.

"Oh no, never in a high-ranking Brahmin family. I heard her wailing before the servants carried her rickshaw to the main house. The house is a large hundred-year-old sandstone, a family of great wealth."

Father cleared his throat. "The servants set a bright yellow gold-trimmed rickshaw in front of me. The lady pushed her hand through the red curtain. The brother wanted me to look at her hand and make a diagnosis. I asked questions, but I couldn't understand anything because she cried while she talked."

"How are you supposed to help if you can't examine your patient?" Ida said.

"The brother explained that her eyes felt like sand scraping across them."

"I probed more, and when the brother told me her eyelids had turned inside out, I knew it was too late."

"What agony." Marmee clipped a thread.

Father nodded. "My diagnosis is trachoma, but that's a guess. I demonstrated to the brother how to administer eye drops. The drops will soothe her eyes, but she'll still have pain. Eventually, she'll go blind."

"Is there anything you can do?" Ida fisted her hand. Outside the heavy rain drowned out the night-time sounds.

He shook his head. "She's probably had untreated conjunctivitis numerous times as a child. Her eyelids scarred. Now the eyelashes scrape against her eyes."

"I'll pray for her," Ida said.

"Too many people in this area go blind," Marmee said. "If they'd come to the dispensary when they first get an eye infection, Father could give them the eye drops to cure it."

"Why don't they come right away?"

"Superstitions." Father shrugged. "They believe that one of their gods has willed it."

"Traditions," Marmee said. "The Brahmin and Hindu women in *zenanas*, the private living quarters for women, only see the other women in their family. In most situations, the matriarch relies on old remedies to cure illnesses."

"Some of those remedies create bigger problems. I've seen patients with cayenne rubbed in their eyes, even broken glass." Father stood and took Marmee's hand. "Come here, lovely wife. Time to settle for the night." Father helped her out of the chair, walked her to the door, and unhooked a lantern from the wall.

Ida slapped her journal shut and followed Marmee and Father. She'd written drivel about how she missed shopping, dancing, and tennis matches. Too many people here suffered to worry about a social life in America. Her life was luxurious compared to women in Vellore. Every job she did at the mission—even cleaning the godown—gave her great satisfaction after a hard day's work. The whining must stop.

Ida turned the oil lantern off and caught up to Father and Marmee on the veranda. "Father?" She grabbed his arm. "Can't you insist the men allow you to give their wives medical care? It's not right for someone to suffer all their life, when a few drops of medicine could prevent permanent damage."

"We have to accept the ways of the people here." Father took a deep breath. "It's a burden to know there's suffering and not be allowed to help, but I know specifically what to pray about. Don't underestimate the need for prayer."

Ida watched outside her bedroom door while her parents walked to their room. "I understand why you came now." The pelting rain drowned out her whisper.

CHAPTER 9

In November, Ida, Henry, Cousin Lew, and her parents celebrated Thanksgiving at the bungalow. A week later, Marmee helped Ida organize the supplies for a trip to the remote villages.

Ida wanted to go on this trip as much as a child wanted Christmas morning to arrive. She pointed to the crates, boxes, and baskets covering a quarter of the veranda. "The ponies may not be able to pull the wagon once we pack everything."

Marmee stood beside Ida with a pencil and pad of paper, checking off the packing list. "That's the reason we send Souri to set up camp a day in advance. There's not enough room for you, Father, Uncle Jared, and Dixie to travel along with the supplies. Between Father and Uncle Jared, they'll see hundreds of patients in the next sixteen days." She turned to Souri, who walked back and forth from the veranda to the wagon loading rice bags and grain.

"I forgot to explain the baby baptisms." Marmee put her list on the wagon and lifted a cloth covering the top of a basket.

Ida peered in the basket. "The baptismal gowns."

"Before your Father baptizes a baby, slip the gown on." Marmee pulled a gown from the basket, opened the drawstring at the bottom of the gown, and pretended to slide a baby into it. "The mothers rub coconut oil over the newborns, and the babies are slippery." Marmee placed the garment back in the basket and covered it. "The gown makes it easier to hold the baby."

"I'm nervous about holding a baby." Ida bit her lip. "What if I drop it?"

"Use both of your hands, and the mother will help you." Marmee turned toward the cart and watched Souri. "Do you see the crate Souri is loading? Those are the tracts. Please pass them around while your Father preaches."

"Why do we give a tract to villagers if they can't read?"

Marmee gave Ida her I'm-glad-you-asked-that-question smile. "The people like to look at the pictures in the tracts. You can also read the tract to them. You'll be traveling to reach the Festival of Lights. There will be thousands of people from the cities on pilgrimage for the festival. Most of them can read, especially the men." Marmee scurried around the wagon.

"After a full year of Tamil lessons, I still don't speak fluently."

"Patience, dear. Remember, 'study to show thyself approved.' When your Father and I moved to India, we were newlyweds. I worried, too, but reading, writing, and eventually speaking in Tamil became as natural as English." Marmee reached for a tract and handed it to Ida. "In case you have trouble with the reading in Tamil, I packed a sample written in English. Study it, and you'll know what the tract says."

The trip should be a success with Marmee's meticulous planning and directions. Ida carried another crate to the wagon. She caught Marmee's attention and then pretended to drop the box.

"Careful," Marmee gasped, "there's glass—"

Ida laughed and balanced the crate in one hand like a waiter carrying a tray. "Don't worry. This crate must have the bandages in it."

By the time Ida and Souri finished packing the wagon, the sun left Ida soaked with perspiration. She smiled to herself, thinking about the coppersmith bird and the hoopoe that she recognized by their songs. Other than the array of year-round flowers that bloomed in India, she loved the birds the most.

Souri hung cooking pots, lanterns, rope, and a shovel on the front of the wagon.

"I don't see any space for the tents," Ida said.

"My brother is at the stable harnessing the bullock cart. He'll carry the tents," Souri said.

"One more item." Marmee held a jug of water. "Here's your clean water, Souri. We don't want you sick."

That evening, Father and Ida waited at the train station in Tindivanam for Uncle Jared and Dixie. At least a dozen other men milled around the dusty ground waiting for the train. The train ground to a stop over the metal rails, spewing steam. Through a cloud of dust, her cousin and Uncle walked out.

Even with a hat on, Dixie didn't reach Uncle Jared's shoulder. Among the crowd, her beautiful cousin looked so young. If she didn't know Dixie was twenty-six, Ida would guess she was a teenager.

"Dixie." Ida hurried and wrapped her arms around her cousin's shoulders.

"Ida." Uncle Jared's gray beard reached his stomach.

Ida jumped at the sound of her uncle's booming voice. "Uncle Jared." She stepped toward her uncle, her heart pounding in her chest.

Uncle Jared took her hand and shook it. "Ida Sophia Scudder. I'm glad you realized you're a part of the Scudder family tradition of missionaries. Your parents need you."

"Sir?" Ida straightened her shoulders. Uncle Jared and his strong opinions. How dare he expect her to give up everything to carry on a family legacy of missionaries. She had plans. Uncle Jared's words pricked her like a thorn bush. "I'm here, aren't I?" Ida said.

Dixie tugged Ida's hand away. "Shall we find some shade?" The two walked to the far end of the platform and chatted. Uncle Jared and Father waited while the porters unloaded the trunks and suitcases.

"Ida, I want to hear all about your first year in Tindivanam," Dixie said.

"The most remarkable part of my first year is Marmee's recovery." Ida smiled and shook her head. "I truly thought I was traveling to my mother's funeral."

"Yes, we've prayed for her every day," Dixie said.

"I know." Ida stood silent for a few moments, reflecting on the past year, remembering how sick Marmee had been. "I was scared and angry before I got to India. When I saw Marmee so weak, I determined to do anything I could. We've stayed so busy, I forgot how upset I was at first. God performed a miracle."

Five minutes later, Father waved his hat at Ida. "We're ready."

When they returned to the mission, Marmee and Salomi served a lentil soup for supper. Uncle Jared blessed the food, praising God for Marmee's health and asking for her safety while they left her at the mission. He prayed for the mission in Vellore. He prayed about their trip. Ida opened one eye and checked the clock on the desk. He prayed longer than anyone she'd ever heard.

Ten minutes later, Ida sighed when he ended with a loud "Aaaaaaaaaa-men."

While Father and Uncle Jared discussed the trip to the villages, Ida noticed the concern in Father's eyes. He tilted his head toward Marmee. "Sixteen days is a long time to leave you alone."

"Henry is checking on me. He's also bringing the older boys from the school to help with chores," Marmee said.

"Ida should stay here. Dixie can assist us," Uncle Jared said.

Ida gulped. The bite of bread balled in her throat. No. She was looking forward to the trip. Why did Uncle Jared think he was to speak for her?

Ida caught Dixie's eyes dart between their two fathers.

"You are in God's hands." Father patted Marmee's hands. He turned to Uncle Jared. "If I leave Ida behind, I'd show God what a lack of faith I had in Him. Marmee's healthy." Father wiped his mouth with a napkin, stood, and pushed his chair in.

Ida's mouth muscles twitched. Stifling a laugh, she turned her head to hide the smile creeping over her face. She didn't want to disrespect her uncle.

Dixie yawned. "We've had a long day on the train. I'm ready for bed, but I'd like a tour of the mission first."

"Follow me," Ida said. She was more than ready to escape Uncle Jared. Ida walked Dixie around the property, showing her the stables, boys' school, and church.

"My father definitely thinks like the older generation, but he means well. You'll see," Dixie said, following Ida to the bedroom. Dixie opened her satchel, found her comb, and ran it through her dark curls.

"What do you want to do with your life?" Ida said with the hope that maybe she and Dixie would go back to America at the same time.

"I want to be a Bible teacher and travel to the remote villages in India and live with the families."

When she was younger, Ida wanted to follow in Dixie's footsteps, but not anymore. Why was Dixie determined to stay in India? Ida wrote that question in her journal and pondered the answer before falling asleep.

Early the next morning, the family ate a quick breakfast of bread, spread with mango chutney. Uncle Jared and Father packed their medical bags and readied the wagon.

Ida and Father hugged Marmee goodbye and took the wagon to the train station. Within an hour, the four boarded the train in Tindivanam. After a half-day's travel, Souri met them at the train stop with the pony cart. Banyan trees lined the path to the village another five miles away.

Thirty minutes later, Ida, her father, uncle, and cousin reached the village. Souri stopped the cart beneath the shade of a tamarind tree, where he'd pitched their tents, and gave the ponies a bucket of water.

People poured from their huts like water spilling out of a cup and gathered around Father and Uncle Jared. Naked toddlers held their mother's hands. School-aged children chased each other, while the adults settled under the tree. Everyone held glass bottles of different shapes and sizes.

"Why are they holding the empty bottles?" Ida unpacked the box of bandages and gauze.

Dixie arranged Uncle Jared's medical equipment at the end of the bullock cart. "If they are prescribed medicine, they use the bottle to keep it in."

Ida spotted an oleander bush in bloom. She rushed over, gathered an armful of blooms, and came back to Dixie, who was assisting Uncle Jared. Ida tucked a sprig of pale pink oleander in Dixie's hair. "You look lovely."

"Take the flowers out of your hair," Uncle Jared said. "We're not here to model frivolousness."

"As you wish." Dixie carefully plucked the flowers from her hair and handed the oleanders to a little girl.

Ida blew out a long breath. Father unfurled a white cotton bed sheet and slid the tools from a velvet-lined pouch and laid his equipment across it. Ida walked over next to him. "What's my job?"

"Spread the surgical knives out in order of size." He handed her a leather pouch. "I like your bouquet," he whispered.

Ida smirked. After organizing the surgical tools, she put her hands on her hips and stomped back to the oleander bush. The shape of their blooms made Ida think of the dogwoods back in Massachusetts at Northfield Seminary.

A few minutes later, Ida returned with her head covered in flowers. She stood against a tree, rubbing her hands over the flowery wig, and watched while Father and Uncle Jared tended to the natives.

Souri directed the villagers into a line. "Move back." He held his arm out to barricade the anxious people from swarming her father and uncle. Instead of one person at a time, it appeared an entire family came with each patient. Dixie made her way through the crowd, wiping babies' noses, administering drops in eyes for people with sore eyes, or applying salve on itchy skin.

The sun blazed overhead against a blue sky, wilting Ida and the flowers on her head. A flower dropped from her hair and fell to the ground. After watching her Father from a distance, she walked over to him to get a better look. Father lanced a boil on a woman's leg. Uncle Jared stitched a cut on a boy's arm. Neither of them noticed her.

Ida didn't know what to do with herself. She didn't belong in this village with goats and dogs and hordes of loud people milling around. She certainly couldn't tolerate another minute of Uncle Jared. In the morning, she'd ask Souri to accompany her back to Tindivanam so she could go back to help Marmee.

CHAPTER 10

Deep laughter brought Ida's attention back from her thoughts.

Uncle Jared stood, wiped the sweat off his brow, and held his stomach.

"What's so funny, Jared?" Father said.

"John, you have your hands full with this daughter of yours. If she knows how to draw a belly laugh out of an old man like me, I think she's capable of anything she sets her mind on."

Ida sauntered over, pretending she was royalty. "Flowers make a wonderful hat." She tapped her head with both hands and yanked a wilted flower out. "For you, Uncle Jared."

Uncle Jared slid the flower in his beard, plucked another one from Ida's head, and stuck it in Father's beard. "Your wig's thirsty."

Ida burst into laughter. "Maybe you're not near the grouch I thought you were after all." Ida stiffened and covered her mouth.

Uncle Jared ignored her comment and began an examination on a man holding his jaw. The line of people waiting to see the doctors wound so far through the village Ida couldn't see the end. Beside her, Father stitched a man's cut on his hand.

"Ida, hand me the tongs and a cotton ball. I need to extract a tooth," Uncle Jared said.

Ida found the equipment on the cart and passed it to Uncle Jared. "Hold his head steady for me until I finish." Uncle Jared clamped the dental forceps around the man's tooth.

The man, squirmed, grunted, and threw his head side to side.

"Hold him still."

Ida tightened her hands on the man's head, wishing she could squeeze her eyes shut.

Uncle Jared twisted and yanked. "Got it!" He held the rotten tooth with the forceps. "Staunch that bleeding with the cotton. Quickly now, girl." Uncle Jared growled his orders and stood over Ida like a bear watching a cub. "Slide it right on the wound."

After tending to the patient, Ida walked back to the cart and sighed. "I think I'll find Dixie and help her." Uncle Jared grunted something she didn't understand.

Across a field of sweet potato vines, a flock of crows squawked at each other. Ida followed the path to the huts and found Dixie visiting a mother. "Dixie, why don't you rest? I'll take over," Ida said.

Dixie cradled a newborn in her arms and nodded towards the young woman sitting beside her. "This is Chandini. Would you like to hold Chandini's baby? Cradle your arms, and I'll pass her to you."

Ida did as Dixie instructed and received the baby from her cousin. The infant—a girl—smelled of coconut oil. Ida watched the baby's brown eyes follow hers. She gave the baby her finger to grasp. "What's her name?" Ida said.

"Chandini is waiting to baptize her before she names her."

"*Dori san avaḻai peyariṭu.* Mrs. John name her," Chandini said.

"Mrs. John is not here. She's been sick. I'm Dori san's daughter."

Chandini nodded. "You name her."

"The Christian families want biblical names for their children," Dixie said.

By late afternoon, Uncle Jared and Father finished seeing patients. Dixie and Ida gathered the medical equipment and cleaned it. After washing, Dixie dried each piece and Ida laid them in the velvet-lined case.

Uncle Jared and Father tied up their waist-length beards, loosened their ties, and with Bibles in hand, walked to the mud-hut church. Ida and Dixie gathered the tracts and baptism gowns and followed.

Dixie stood at the entrance, handing out tracts as people arrived for the church service. Ida waited in the front for the baptisms to begin. After both Uncle Jared and Father preached, the mothers lined up to have their babies baptized.

Ida's heart pumped so hard she could feel it against her chest. *Don't worry. You won't drop the baby.* Sitting on the mat, she slid a gown over each baby's head.

Chandini was next. Ida kissed the baby's forehead, relieved to have the job done. "This beautiful girl's name shall be Esther." She handed the bundle to Father.

"Little Miss Esther, I baptize you in the name of the Father, the Son, and the Holy Spirit. Amen." Father dipped water from an earthen vase and sprinkled the water on the baby's head.

After the service, Dixie joined a group of women to talk with them. Ida waited nearby in front of a cactus hedge.

An old man whacked the ground with his cane.

Ida's heart jumped. Was he going to hit her?

"Step away from the cactus."

Ida stared at him. Until something caught her eye, and she took a step back.

"Don't move. There's a cobra!" he yelled.

Ida stopped mid-step and screamed. She put her foot down as dainty as a ballerina.

"The snake is frightened. Stand still."

"The snake is frightened?" Ida said, her voice shrill. "I'm terrified."

"I'm a snake handler," he said. The barefoot, bare-chested man leaned forward. The cobra hissed and slithered in his direction. "It's ready to strike."

Please, dear God, get us out of here alive.

CHAPTER 11

Ida's muscles tensed. Her eyes darted from snake to snake handler and back to the snake. Her heart drummed so hard she worried the snake would feel the vibrations.

The snake handler thumped his stick on the ground again. The snake hissed. Two other men approached from either side of the snake. The villagers circled around. Children shimmied their way to the front and sat cross-legged on the ground, as if watching a show. Ida expected complete silence and scared people. Instead the audience jabbered, some yelled directions, and the children screeched when the snake moved.

The snake handler crouched about six feet away. Back, forward, and sideways, he dodged the cobra's movements. He flexed his hand, cupped his hand, and pointed two fingers up and down.

The handler moved closer, taunting the snake with his hand movements. The cobra slithered toward the man. Two feet in the air, the cobra held its neck erect.

A wide black band marked the bottom of the cobra's throat.

"Watch out. It's going to strike." Ida pressed her closed fist against her lips.

"The snake doesn't see me as a threat when my hand is in this position." The snake handler kept his posture crouched and talked to Ida with his eyes glued on the snake. "See how calm it is."

Her pulse pounded all the way through her neck. *Dear God in heaven, You promised to protect. Please keep this brave man safe.*

From the left, a teenage boy stepped out of the crowd and slid the handler a round basket with a lid.

Ida moved sideways to get farther away, and the snake's neck whipped around. As fast as her heart pounded, the snake handler tapped the ground with the cane. The snake slithered back toward him.

On the right an elderly man stepped from the crowd into the opening between Ida and the snake handler. "Gentle," he called directions to the handler. The older man watched intently. "Don't make a quick movement."

The handler held the stick in one hand, waved his other hand at the cobra's head, and talked to the cobra like he was coaxing a child.

The snake stretched itself forward.

"Wait, wait, wait." The elderly man directed the snake handler. "Hold steady. Now!"

The handler pressed the tail with his foot, and then held the snake right behind its head with his stick. The elder man sprung forward, opened the basket, tilted it on the side, and bounced back out of the way.

The crowd ooh-oohed. The kids covered their mouths and leaned their heads and shoulders back, as if the snake might come their way.

Ida held her breath.

Inch by inch the handler moved the stick further back on the snake's body, while the snake slithered into the basket. He lifted the stick while the cobra curled its upper body into the basket. The crowd silenced. The old man leapt over to the basket and pushed the lid on the cobra's head, while the handler pushed the snake's tail inside. The teenage boy darted beside the two other men and opened a canvas bag. The eldest man slid the basket inside and tied it tight. The handler grabbed the bag and held it in the air.

Ida let out a long sigh but didn't move until she watched the elder man take the bag and leave. While the crowd hooped and clapped and whistled, she shivered all over.

The snake handler motioned for her. Ida checked the ground before she walked over to him. "I was so frightened."

"Last week seven people died in this village from cobra bites."

"If you hadn't been here—" Ida stopped. *God was here.* "I'm so grateful."

Dixie ran to Ida and led her to the wagon.

Uncle Jared and Father knelt on the ground. "Our great Creator, we thank thee for saving our Ida," Uncle Jared said.

After a pause, Father prayed. "We thank thee for the men and their wisdom to remove the cobra."

Ida dropped to her knees beside Father. Tears seeped from behind her closed eyelids. "Thank you for guiding the snake handlers." She stopped praying and watched Uncle Jared.

Father held Ida's hand and helped her stand. "Stick close to me the rest of the day."

By evening the village had prepared a feast for Ida and her relatives. Beneath a palm tree, village women spread mats over the ground. The air smelled smoky from the trench fires where rice simmered in big, black pots.

Ida and Dixie found a spot and sat cross-legged in front of a banana-leaf plate. A woman mounded rice and curry on the leaves. Ida scooped her food with her hand like everyone else. "The curry tastes spicier than it smells." She waved her hand in front of her, trying to cool off her mouth. When everyone finished eating, the women set bamboo containers and bowls out.

An older Indian woman hunched on her knees sat beside Ida. She raised the lid on the bamboo container. "Curds to cool your tongue." She lifted a small bowl and sipped. "The pepper water cools the spices too."

Ida leaned toward Dixie and muttered. "Pepper water? This looks like a soup."

"The pepper water is a soup made with tomatoes, lentils, and black peppercorns," Dixie said, "but they call it water." With both hands she held the bowl to her lips and sipped.

"Eat the leaf." The old woman rubbed her belly and flashed a toothless smile at Ida. "It's good for your tummy."

Dixie tore a section of the leaf and nibbled on it. Ida wiped the rice off the banana leaf and rolled it around her head and held her arms out. "Ta-da. I'm a princess."

The old woman cackled.

Dixie opened her eyes wide. "Ida, you're such a cutup."

Ida winked, then rolled the leaf in a tube, and dipped it in the curds. She held it like it was a banana and licked the curds off the leaf. "Tastes like sour cream but better. And my tongue is cooler." Then Ida painted a white mustache above her lips with the curds.

The older woman clapped.

That night, Ida bathed behind a thin reed shelter. Imagining how good a shower would feel when she made it back to the mission, she dipped her washcloth in the *parnee*, a small cup of water. On the way back to the tent, she checked the distance between the cactus hedge and their tents. They camped a field away, but Ida wished Souri would have changed the camp's location after the cobra incident.

By the time she returned to the tent, Dixie had fallen asleep. The tent was hardly big enough for both cots, but Ida squeezed in quietly. The only sounds were the constant chirp of crickets.

Several times throughout the night Ida jerked to an upright position and cupped her ears to make sure she didn't hear a hiss. Her muscles tensed, ready to flee. *It's only the insects.* She sighed and settled back onto the cot.

Before the first rays of light, Ida got up to dress.

Dixie rolled over, sat up, and yawned. "Ida, are you sick? Why are you wearing all those petticoats?"

"Protection against snake bites."

Dixie snickered. "You're more likely to die from heat than a snake. Take off those petticoats."

Ida buttoned her high-collared shirt. "I'm wearing two until we leave this campsite." Ida hunched down and slipped out of the tent.

Father, Uncle Jared, and Souri were awake and preparing to leave for the next village. Uncle Jared stood on the wagon and boxed the medical supplies. Souri carried grain to the ponies. Father left to check on a patient. Some of the villagers waited near the campsite. Dixie and Ida spent the next thirty minutes reading and passing out more tracts. Ida felt more comfortable reading the tracts than when she first arrived at the village.

Ready to leave the village by eight o'clock, they followed the dirt road west toward Tiruvannamalai. Thorny shrubs leaned over the road and scraped the wagon wheels. The road turned hilly and thickened with travelers heading west. Wagons, bullock carts, bicyclists, and people carried on palanquins made their way to the temple. Many hikers carried a long stick across their shoulders with brass pots balanced on both ends.

"What's in the pots?" Ida said.

"Ghee or camphor. They're taking it to burn in the copper cauldron at the temple for the festival," Dixie said.

Lush green trees and shrubs covered the hills. When they reached Tiruvannamalai, Souri parked the wagon on a hillside in a clearing as close to a temple as he could.

Ida climbed out of the wagon, followed by Dixie, Father, and Uncle Jared. The smell of eucalyptus, coconut, and sweat wafted through the air.

Father spread a sheet out for patients and opened his doctor bag. Souri invited people around them to see the doctor. Uncle Jared tied his beard, climbed onto the wagon, and began preaching.

Ida stared at the view. Temples towered high into the sky like white skyscrapers.

"Come on, Dixie, let's walk closer."

Ida and Dixie shimmied their way through a sea of people. Men blew conch shell horns. Another set of men with shaved heads sat in front of the temple and chanted.

"The men are Shiva devotees. They cover their body in red powder and sandalwood paste for Shiva, a Hindu god," Dixie said.

Ida and Dixie watched while hundreds of people walked to the temple doors and left their pots of ghee and camphor. A group of girls danced. Their silver and brass bracelets, necklaces, and headbands tingled with each turn.

"They're *devadasis*, or girls who give their lives to the temple," Dixie said.

"They're beautiful."

"Unfortunately, the girls don't live at the temple by choice. They are given to the temple," Dixie said. "Like high-caste Hindu women living their lives in zenanas, the temple girls don't experience life beyond the temple gates."

"I feel so sad for them."

Dixie sighed. "Me too."

Ida and her cousin walked among throngs of people, while Dixie explained the cultural practices. "The people have traveled hundreds of miles to see the cauldron light up. They believe the gods light the fire, and once they see the light, their salvation is assured," Dixie said.

They stopped to watch men leading an elephant with a double-decker palanquin on its back. Stacked like the layers of a cake, the palanquin was painted gold and scarlet with a statue of Shiva on top.

Ida and Dixie returned an hour later, and Uncle Jared was still preaching.

A crowd circled around him yelling, "*Govinda. Govinda.*"

"What are they yelling?" Ida said to Dixie.

"They're chanting the name of a Hindu god."

"They're taunting him." Ida put her hands on her hips.

Uncle Jared stepped off the wagon, his shirt soaked from perspiration. He wiped the sweat dripping off his face with a handkerchief.

Father climbed onto the wagon with his Bible and began to preach.

The crowd continued chanting. Father preached for over an hour and ignored the hecklers. Then Uncle Jared took over. They alternated all afternoon between preaching and seeing patients.

By dinnertime Ida and Dixie found a shady spot at the edge of the hill overlooking the temple. Ida spread a tablecloth on the ground, and Dixie unpacked their food. Uncle Jared and Father stopped working and joined them.

Ida cleared her throat. "I wondered why you continued preaching while the crowd jeered." She glanced at Father and then Uncle Jared.

Uncle Jared straightened his back and set his plate on the ground. "Scudders are not cowards. Scudders run into obstacles not from them. And you know the story of your grandfather?" He looked at Father.

"She knows how her grandfather left a medical practice in America to come to India." Father rolled his flat bread, *chapati*, and dipped it in kidney-bean curry.

"And I know my grandmother, Harriet, bore ten children and my father is the youngest."

"Our father," Uncle Jared cleared his throat, "didn't have a horse and wagon. He traveled by foot into the Mysore forests, escaping wild animals."

Uncle Jared continued the story with sound effects and detailed descriptions. Ida could imagine the weather, taste the food, and feel the emotions in her mind that her grandparents endured. "You're a marvelous historian," Ida said. "Why don't you tell stories when you preach?"

"When you take over the mission, you can deliver God's word the way you see fit." He leaned his head forward. "Do you think your grandparents would want us to concede to hecklers?"

"No," Ida said in a subdued tone. "Scudders don't quit." She stood and wiped the crumbs off her skirt.

"Look toward the temples," Dixie said. "*Kathihai Teepam*. The Festival of Lights."

The sunset turned the sky to a deep purple. On a distant hilltop, a flare of yellow light hit the skyline.

"The priests fill the ghee and camphor into a gigantic copper cauldron and light the cotton wicks," Dixie said.

A red sphere highlighted the hillside behind the temples. From the valley below, the thousands of visitors shouted. Ida and Dixie watched while the giant flame burned for the next hour.

"Fascinating," Ida said. How could people fall on their knees to worship a huge torch like it held power? Uncle Jared and Father were right to share God's story, but standing on the back of a wagon yelling wasn't the way she wanted to share God's story. Why didn't Father and Uncle Jared just talk to their patients about God while they examined them?

No matter what her family did in the past, she wasn't about to continue the legacy of Scudder missionaries. What was she going to do with her life? She was at a complete loss. She crossed her arms, certain her plans didn't include preaching and practicing medicine.

CHAPTER 12

Sixteen days later, Ida arrived home exhausted from the trip, more thankful to be home than ever. Even cleaning the godown didn't fluster her after the snake scare. If she ever saw another cobra, Ida hoped it would be in a snake charmer's basket.

One evening, Ida sat at her desk to write to friends back home. A lizard scampered up the wall and disappeared into the thatch, splattering dirt down onto Ida's desk. She swept the dirt off and opened the box of stationery.

Dear Annie,

In a month we are moving to a much larger town, Vellore. The town is seventy miles from Tindivanam and closer to Madras, a large city. How I miss a city! I'm sure I've lost touch with the latest fashions.

A rustling outside caught her attention. Ida dropped her pen and peered through the window. The full moon lit the veranda. A carriage stopped, and a man stepped out. Nothing out of the ordinary here. Visitors often showed up at different hours of the night for Father's help.

Ida opened her door. "Can I help you, sir?"

The man bowed. Ida recognized him as a Brahmin gentleman by his dress. He wore the clothes of a high-ranking Hindu. The three-stranded white thread, symbolizing twice-born, hung across his shoulder.

"Yes, Ammal." He spoke in English. "My wife. She is in childbirth and is not doing well. She will not live. I hear you are from America. Please, can you come to assist her?"

"Excuse me while I get the doctor." Ida rushed over to her parents' bedroom door and banged.

"Yes?" Father said in a tired voice.

"There's a Brahmin man who needs a doctor. It's urgent."

In his night clothes, he opened the door a crack. "I'll be right out."

Ida closed the door and turned. The Brahmin man stood inches away, blocking her path. "No man has ever looked upon my wife, and no man ever will."

Ida lifted the lantern to see the man's face. He glared at her, his brows furrowed. "But you want to save your wife's life, don't you?"

"Another man is not allowed to see my wife." He crossed his arms.

"I'm the doctor's daughter, not the doctor." Ida studied his face. If only she could make him understand and ease his anger, maybe he'd make an allowance to save his wife.

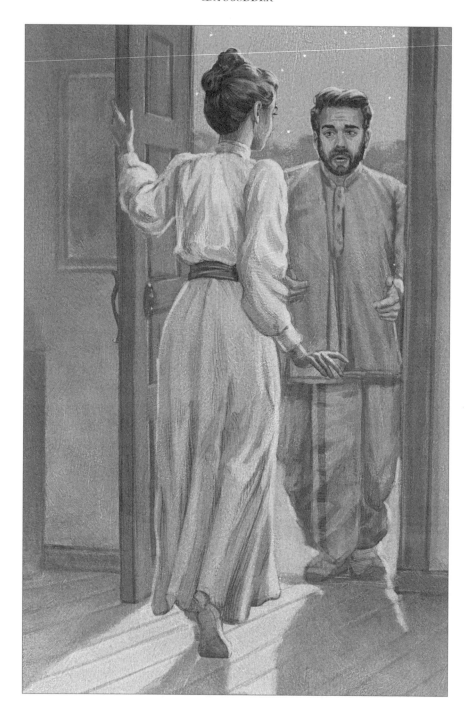

Ida pressed into the wall. "You said she was dying. Your wife will need an operation to save the baby."

Father opened the door. Ida and the Brahmin stood there in a stare down. She turned and put her hand on Father's shoulder. "This is Dr. Scudder. He is the only doctor here."

The Brahmin scrutinized Father like he was a monster. "My wife will manage alone. If her fate is death, then so it must be." He turned and walked to the carriage without another word.

Ida stepped toward the retreating man.

Father grabbed her shoulders. "There is nothing we can do."

"How can he just leave?" Her voice pitched an octave higher. "His wife is dying." She reached back for the door.

"Remember, we must respect his decision."

Ida looked up at the stars that wallpapered the night sky. The big dipper hung like it waited for stardust to fill its bucket. She sighed. *God, please save his wife.*

Ida rushed back to her room, bolted the door shut, and sunk into the desk chair. Her mind was too agitated to sleep. *Please, Lord, send him back for Father before it is too late.*

She crumpled the letter to Annie and dipped her pen in the inkwell to begin another one. Ida peered out the window at a faint light. A lantern swayed on the front of a carriage. Ida jumped up. *He's returned for Father.*

The moment the carriage stopped, Ida burst outside. "I'm so glad you changed your mind." Ida held a lantern to illuminate the man's face and gasped.

A Muslim gentleman with a long-buttoned coat and a white brocade cap stood in front of her, not the Brahmin. "Salaam. I am sorry to disturb you at such a late hour. My wife is a girl of fourteen. The barber woman came to deliver the baby, but she said to leave my wife to die."

How can I tell another husband I can't save his wife? Ida felt her blood drain from her face. Again Ida explained she wasn't the doctor.

The Muslim man refused Father the same as the Brahmin man.

She stomped back to her room and dropped her head on the desk. What could be worse than this living nightmare? *Dear Lord. This is too awful. Please, don't let them die.*

Ida abandoned the letter, turned down the light, and lay on top of the covers, trying to push the horrible thoughts away. At 2:00 a.m., after tossing and bobbing around in her bed like a float lost at sea, she got up and went to finish writing to Annie. From outside, someone clearing his throat caught Ida's attention. She grabbed the light and walked to the door, not confident it was either the Brahmin or Muslim. But maybe. She could only hope.

Ida swung the door open. A Mudalier man, with his huge turban edged in a gold band, stood in front of her.

"You're Kamla's father, aren't you?" Ida knew his daughter from the school for girls run by the mission. "Is Kamla sick?" Ida felt her stomach wrench.

The man dropped to his knees and bowed at her feet. "*Illai,* no. Kamla is not sick. Her mother is in great jeopardy with a delivery. Please come."

The words blurred in Ida's head like the tears blurring her vision. Just like the previous husbands, the man stood, took a moment to thank Ida, but dashed to his carriage alone.

Ida watched the night turn from black to the morning sky. In the distance, the blare of horns and the beat of a tom-tom boomed through the air. Her heart dropped with each beat.

Ida sprinted to the stone wall beyond the tamarind thicket that surrounded the mission and peeked over the edge. She had to see for herself if the funeral was for one of the mothers. Souri followed her.

Men in white turbans passed with their tom-toms. Behind the drummers a group carried small plantain trees and swayed the green fronds. Mourners followed the wicker coffin covered in a red cloth. The line stretched as long as three train cars. Near the end, Kamla walked beside the pallbearers.

Kamla. Too young to have lost her mother.

Twenty to thirty relatives at the end of the procession chanted and wailed.

"Ammal," Souri said, "What is the trouble?"

"A Brahmin and a Muslim gentleman also visited here last night. Both of their wives were in labor." She described the visitors as fast as she could speak. "Can you find their homes? I must know if the wives are alive. Maybe there's time."

Souri nodded. "There is a way to find out. Let me get the pony."

Light filtered above the tree line. "Hurry." She rushed to the bungalow knowing only one choice

75

remained. Inside her room, she hurled herself to the rug, bent on her knees.

"Jesus." Ida dabbed her eyes with a handkerchief. "Three times I awoke to a voice. What is it you're trying to tell me?" Over and over the same thought returned—*the women of India need a woman doctor.* Tears trickled down her cheeks.

A knock interrupted Ida's prayer. She sprung up and whipped the door open. Souri stood on the veranda.

"I found the families, Ammal."

"Tell me. Is there still time to save the two wives?"

"The wives . . ." He shook his head. "They died."

Ida clutched her stomach. "Three mothers. All dead."

CHAPTER 13

Ida's eyes pooled with tears. "Why did they have to die?"

Souri took Ida by the arm and led her to the bedroom door. "Please, go rest before chota is served." He stopped on the porch. "Death is part of life, isn't it?"

"Why is *unnecessary* death a part of life?" Ida unlocked her door. "Those mothers could have been saved if . . . if only the women had a doctor."

Ida slipped under the covers and attempted sleep, but her mind wouldn't shut off. *You must help.* She turned on her stomach and covered her head with the pillow, but the thought persisted . . . *you can care for the women.*

Ida sat straight up. Where were these thoughts coming from? No, she couldn't give up her plans. Why . . . now . . . did the dream of lobster bisque, fancy dresses, and summer dances sound shallow?

"God, is it you speaking?" Ida looked upward. Her voice was barely a whisper, her breath only short wisps. *What can I do for the women?* Ida grabbed her Bible and prayed.

For several minutes, Ida read through 1 Samuel 3. *Here I am, Lord.* Ida knelt beside her bed, leaned her head against the mattress and listened to her thoughts.

Ida prayed, "Speak, Lord, thy servant hears."

The early morning sounds of people beginning their day filtered through the window. Wooden wheels ground against the dirt streets, drivers called "Hinh, hinh" to their bullocks. And another tom-tom. Another funeral.

Ida heard a rustle outside followed by a voice. "Chota."

She rose to open the door.

Salomi set the chota on the desk.

Ida thanked Salomi and opened the Bible back to reread 1 Samuel. She wasn't prepared to face the day. When she reached verse nine, she read aloud. " 'Therefore Eli said unto Samuel, Go, lie down: and it shall be, if he call thee, that thou shalt say, Speak LORD; for they servant heareth.' "

A rush of excitement ran through her. Why couldn't she be a doctor? A female physician is what the wives needed. Ida turned her head toward the ceiling. *God, if you need me, I will serve.*

Ida rose, splashed water on her face, dried it, and combed her hair up into a bun. Then she dashed from her room to the office and threw open the door. As she'd expected to see, Marmee sat on the settee reading the Bible. Father stood at his desk, packing his medical bag.

"Father. Marmee." Ida bored her eyes into each one. "I know what I'm supposed to do with my life now."

Marmee tilted her head and looked calm as always. "What is it?"

Father raised his eyebrows. "Go on."

"The women of India need a doctor. I'm going back to America to study medicine to be the doctor the women need."

CHAPTER 14

Ida straightened, clasped her hands together, and waited for Father's and Marmee's reaction. She watched each nuance in their expressions.

Teary-eyed, Father blew his nose in his handkerchief and then embraced Ida. "I've always hoped one of my children would choose medicine." He stepped back and looked at Marmee.

"The way you attended to me when I was sick made me think the medical field might lure you," Marmee said. "You have a talent, dear, and I'm glad God's awakened your heart to it."

Ida swallowed a lump and blinked back tears. "God awoke me all right. Last night seemed like a Samuel experience for me." She took a deep breath. "What do you mean I have a talent?"

"Not everyone can minister to the sick." Marmee grinned. "You possessed patience when I dealt with pain but didn't treat me like a child."

Ida noticed the medical texts behind the glassed bookshelf. She'd dusted around the books every week.

Opening one of those books to read was never an interest before today. Each volume appeared to be two or three inches thick. The task ahead would be great.

"You have the gift of gentleness and long-suffering—all fruit of the spirit. When I watched you care for Marmee, I was touched," Father said. "God's equipped you for the medical profession."

"You have no idea what your words mean to me," Ida said.

Salomi opened the back door. "Excuse me, Dr. John?" Hot air wafted in the room. "Souri says the pony cart is ready."

Father pulled his pocket watch out of his jacket. "I'm on my way." He lifted his doctor bag, kissed Marmee, and paused beside Ida. "I'd like to hear your story, but I need to leave. We'll talk at supper."

"Certainly, Father." Ida waved goodbye. Watching him leave to visit patients presented a whole new meaning to Ida.

Salomi's maize-colored sari billowed as she picked up the dirty dishes. She balanced the dishes in her arms.

"Ida's decided to be a doctor." Marmee's cheek dimpled with her smile.

"But you are a woman," Salomi said.

Ida pursed her lips. Of course, Salomi couldn't fathom a woman doctor. "I'll go back to America to study."

"I will miss you." Salomi frowned.

"Dear, I'm coming back to India to provide medical care for you and other women who can't see a male doctor."

"God is guiding Ida in the right direction. Even in India, He will find a way for her to serve," Marmee said.

"I see." Salomi's brown eyes widened and without another question, she headed through the back door to the kitchen.

"People will need time to accept a female doctor." Marmee waved Ida toward the desk. "We need to plan our move to Vellore." She opened the calendar.

"Three months away. I can't wait to tell Dixie my news."

That evening Ida and her parents sat beneath the *punkah* fan on the veranda. Fireflies flickered above the ground.

Father leaned back in the rocker and propped his feet on a stool. "I'm ready to hear your story."

"I know God showed me His plan." Ida continued to share the details of the previous night with Father and Marmee. Her parents listened without interrupting.

"My heart ached for the helpless women. I felt responsible for their deaths, but my presence wouldn't have made any difference. It was a horrible night." She stopped for a moment, lowered her head, and pressed the palm of her hand against her forehead. Marmee rubbed Ida's back. "I want to help the poor women who have no one to go to when they are sick."

Father took a deep breath. "Everything you've shared confirms to me that God used those events to show you your life's work."

"Father, once I finish school, won't it be wonderful to say 'yes' instead of 'no' to a woman in distress?"

Marmee leaned forward. "It's the most marvelous idea I've ever heard."

"Let's pray." Father grasped Ida's and Marmee's hands, leading them through a prayer of praise and a plea for direction.

Ida kissed them good night, returned to her room, and kneeled by her bed. "Thank you, God for showing me my future and giving me peace. You knew my mission in life all along, didn't you?"

Then Ida lit the lantern, opened her journal, and began to plan.

CHAPTER 15

The summer passed like a whirlwind. Ida wrote a letter for information about enrollment to the Women's Medical College of Pennsylvania. She worried that a medical school might not accept her after a lapse in school. She sealed the envelope and decided fretting wouldn't make any difference. God said not to worry. She determined to pray whenever a doubt niggled at her mind.

Three months later, Ida, Father, and Marmee left Tindivanam and arrived at the Katapidi train station outside of Vellore by late afternoon. The heat wrapped its fiery arms around Ida as she stepped out on the platform. While Ida and Marmee climbed in a cart, Father paid the bullock cart driver to take them to the mission house.

"Do you remember the fort?" Marmee pointed to tall rock walls.

Ida shook her head, wondering why she didn't. "I remembered the temple, but I didn't realize it was inside a fort. What does a seven-year-old girl notice anyway?"

"The fort was built in the sixteenth century. The Hindus abandoned the fort when the Muslims invaded and killed a cow inside it," Marmee said. "The temple is filled with elaborate stone carvings."

"I'd like to take a tour," Ida said.

The bullock chugged past an endless high stone wall surrounding the fort. The driver turned the bullock cart onto a busy road of people walking, rickshaws, carts, wagons, and an occasional cow. "We must be in the middle of the city," Ida said.

They passed the government buildings, a police station, and the English Club. Each building was framed with tidy paths and palm trees. A mile away from town, Ida watched her mother's eyes light up when the mission bungalow came into view.

Stately white columns anchored the veranda. Marmee reached for Ida's hand, smiling as if she were viewing a fine painting. "I have special memories of you and your brothers growing up here. Do you remember your first home in India?"

"The bungalow looks the same as it looked when I was a little girl," Ida said. Rows and rows of hungry children flashed in her mind. "Where did we feed the children the bread and milk every day?" She twisted around looking for the big yard.

"The children sat in the back with their bowls waiting for *congee*." Father pressed his eyes closed for a second, as if pushing back a bad memory. "The 1886 drought left most of southern India starving for two years. The worst drought I've experienced." He patted Ida's knee. "You wanted to give the children your own food."

The driver pulled the yoke and called directions for the bullocks to stop. The cart's wheels crushed twigs on the ground. They stopped underneath a camphor tree across from the bungalow. The camphor's strong odor penetrated the air.

Dixie ran out and down the steps, waving. "I'm so glad you're here." Dixie reached for Marmee to guide her out of the cart. Ida followed.

Banana plants flanked the corner of the bungalow. "You've got bananas ready to pick," Ida said. A stem, weighted by clusters of green bananas, hung near the ground. She sauntered over to the banana tree and glanced back at Dixie and Marmee who watched from the veranda. After studying the ground to make sure the area was clear of cobras, Ida squatted beneath the branch, stretched out her arms, and pretended to balance the bananas on her head.

Ida grunted at the weight. She dipped her body out from underneath the branch, twisted a green banana away from the cluster, and walked back to the bungalow.

Dixie and Marmee laughed.

Ida rotated the end of the banana until it loosened, peeled the skin back, and took a bite. "I settled for one. The branch must weigh a hundred pounds."

Dixie motioned for Ida. "Come inside with us."

"I think I'll take a stroll around the mission." Father waved back.

Dixie opened the door for Ida and Marmee.

"Aunt Julie." Ida greeted her.

"Give me a big hug," Aunt Julie said.

For the first time, Ida noticed how much older Aunt Julia looked than Marmee. Her hair was as white as Uncle Jared's beard.

"Ida, how long has it been since I saw you in Nebraska? Ten? Fifteen years?" Aunt Julia kissed Ida's cheek.

"Twelve years," Ida said. "I was ten."

Aunt Julia clasped Marmee's hands. "Sophia, you were so sick the last time we visited you."

"Recovery was slow, but I'm in good health now." Marmee beamed. "Thanks to Ida and the good Lord."

"Our daughters are indispensable." Aunt Julia grinned, first at Dixie and then at Ida. "Are the two of you ready to tour the mission? We've added some buildings in the back."

"Ready," Ida said.

Dixie and Ida followed Aunt Julia and Marmee. They passed the stable, godown, and smaller cement buildings where the other mission workers lived. Aunt Julia showed them the boys' boarding school, another building for the high-school-aged boys. They stopped at two buildings side-by-side. Flowering bushes grew in front of the buildings and swallowtail butterflies lit on the flowers.

"We have two schools for Hindu girls. With so many attending, we divided the girls into two groups. I split my day between both schools. One class is for the six- to nine-year-old girls and another for ten- to twelve-year-old girls," Dixie said.

"How many students?" Ida said.

"Ninety-three in the younger class and one-hundred and eight in the oldest group. The youngest group goes home at lunch and stays home. The older girls return after lunch for another session."

"I'm surprised at the high enrollment for Hindu girls," Marmee said, looking pleased.

"The Hindu families want the best for their girls, so they're willing to send them to a Christian school for an education," Aunt Julia said.

"I'm glad Ida's here to help. The mission compound has grown so much since we lived here," Marmee said.

Uncle Jared rode the bullock wagon into the stable.

"I see Jared," Aunt Julia said. "Excuse me while I get supper on the table."

The four walked back toward the veranda with Julia and Marmee leading the way. While their mothers went inside, Ida lingered behind to talk to Dixie.

"I almost wish I could go to the States with you, but I have to wait two more years," Ida said.

"Why do you want to go back?" Dixie said.

"I'm going to study medicine," Ida said.

"You're going to be a nurse?"

Ida put her hand on Dixie's shoulder. "I'm going to be a doctor."

Dixie raised her eyebrows. "A doctor? Aren't you going to help your father?"

Ida took a deep breath, trying not to show her disappointment in Dixie's reaction. She hadn't prepared herself for opposition from her cousin. "I believe God's called me to be a doctor for the women who can't leave their zenanas, women who can't allow a man to help them deliver their children. I want to prevent loss of life from minor illnesses simply because a male doctor cannot see or touch them."

"You just preached a sermon," Dixie said. "I apologize. I've never met a female doctor."

"I've applied to the Women's Medical College in Pennsylvania," Ida said.

Father and Uncle Jared approached the veranda. "I hear interesting news about you, Ida," Uncle Jared said. "I know your grandfather would tell you to

follow God's leading, even if it's into unchartered ter-
ritories. May God bless your endeavor." Uncle Jared
patted Ida's shoulder.

"Thank you," Ida's skin tingled. Another
confirmation.

Aunt Julia stuck her head out of the front door.
"Supper." Ida and the remainder of the family followed her to a dining room near the kitchen in the
back of the house. The bungalow was much larger
than the one in Tindivanam. That night after supper,
Aunt Julia, Marmee, and Dixie cleaned up the dishes.
Ida and Father went with Uncle Jared to his office in
the back of the bungalow which winged off into an
L-shape.

"I'll travel to Tindivanam every two weeks to treat
patients until the mission sends a doctor there," Father
said.

"You'll have a strenuous schedule," Uncle Jared
said.

Father shook his head in agreement. "I can't leave
the people in Tindivanam without medical care."

Uncle Jared and Father discussed until bedtime the
management of the mission. That night, Ida was too
excited to sleep. She lay in bed imagining herself ex-
amining patients in Uncle Jared's office.

The next morning, Ida went to the girls' school
with Dixie to meet the students. The girls wore bright
colored saris. Long, dark hair hung in braids down
their backs. Each girl presented Ida with a flower. She
thought the girls were as pretty as the flowers they
lined up to give her.

"Girls, you may play a game of tag while I discuss
your studies with Miss Ida," Dixie said.

"Calisthenics happened to be my best subject in Tindivanam." Ida chuckled. "I'm not confident of any other subjects."

Dixie turned toward the happy voices outside, giving Ida a reassuring look. "The girls are excited to learn. They won't judge your teaching abilities."

"How do you manage both schools?" Ida said.

"My mother teaches as well. We also have several workers who assist you and are also learning English along with the students."

"You've quelled my apprehension," Ida said. She listened to silver anklets jingle while the barefooted girls chased each other. "In my mind, I can already see these girls grown with a husband and children of their own. I pray I'm back in time to be their doctor."

CHAPTER 16

Before sunrise on Monday morning, every member of the Scudder family was up. Ida and her parents bid Uncle Jared, Aunt Julie, and Dixie goodbye. Ida carried coffee, banana, toast, and the morning chota with her to prepare her lessons at the school. Her stomach somersaulted while she listed plans in the journal for the younger class.

Morning Prayers

Math: Add 20 jumping jacks plus 10 ball tosses plus hop on one foot 10 times

English: My teacher's name is Miss Scudder. Play Simon Says and copy Miss Scudder's actions.

Reading: Listen to Exodus 2–3. Act out the story of Moses.

Penmanship: Copy Exodus 3:4. Practice tracing the words in sand outside before copying the verse on the slate.

Now what do I do with the older group? Ida studied the cement wall trying to come up with a clever idea. She wanted her first day in class to be fun and studious. *Why not combine classes in the morning?* She'd ask the older students to tutor the younger students until lunch. That way she'd get an idea of the older girls' skills.

The students trickled in, greeting her with, "Namaste, Ammal Scudder." Each one found a place to sit on a mat and whispered to one another.

A worker from the mission arrived to help. "My name is Mrs. Isaac."

Ida could have hugged her she was so happy to have a helper. She didn't want to frighten Mrs. Isaac. "I'm relieved I don't have to wonder if the girls understand my Tamil. Will you interpret for me, if needed?"

"I will, if you'll help me with my English."

Ida laughed. "I think we'll make a good team."

About midmorning, Ida turned to Mrs. Isaac. "The giggling is enough to tell me they loved Simon Says. There's one problem. I can't remember anyone's name. I'm going to use the slates and have each girl write their name on it. They can hold the slate up when I ask a question, so I can see their name."

"Yes, Ammal Scudder. I will set the slates out for you."

Ida whistled. Silence. The girls looked more like a group of statues than girls. "Did I scare you?"

No one moved. Then one girl raised her hand.

"Yes, dear. What is your name?"

The girl wore a pink sari that reminded Ida of pink geraniums. "My name is Lakshmi. Ammal Scudder, only the police whistle. This is why we stopped."

"Lakshmi, will you explain in Tamil for the girls to not be scared?" Ida waved the girls toward the entrance. "Now girls, after we write our names on the slates, we're going to learn how to whistle."

Before Ida realized it, a year had passed. The Women's Medical College of Pennsylvania approved her application. Now that she knew her exact plans, she wrote to Annie to update her.

Dear Annie,

Life in Vellore is busier than Tindivanam. The Women's Medical College has accepted me based on one criterion. I must pass the state's Regent Exam first. Father and Marmee will leave with me for the United States. See you in the fall of 1894—one more year.

Forever your friend,
Ida

After lunch the next day, Ida returned to the school for the afternoon session with the older girls. The school routine was comfortable to Ida now.

Ida began the class with a song. A half hour later, a man walked into the classroom. "Excuse me, Ammal Scudder. I must speak with my daughter, Lakshmi."

Ida didn't remember seeing her that afternoon. She surveyed the room. "Girls, do you know where Lakshmi is?"

"She walked alone to her village at noon," a student said.

"She never arrived home." Lakshmi's father's jaw tightened. "I will find her." He turned and strode toward the dirt road.

Ida swallowed hard. *Please, God, keep Lakshmi safe.*

Ida couldn't stop her mind from wondering. Was Lakshmi lying beneath a bush dying from a cobra bite? She couldn't be lost, could she? She lived around the corner from the school. Ida tried to act like her age of a twenty-three-year-old adult, but she couldn't pretend she wasn't worried.

"Class, put your slates aside." Ida collected the slates and set them on the shelf by the door.

The room was silent. Their quiet was unnerving. From their wide-eyed stares, the girls were probably worried as much as she was.

Ida motioned to the girls sitting further back in the room, while she settled on a mat in front of the girls. "Scoot close to me." She paused to collect her emotions. "I'm going to pray, dears." Ida bowed her head. "Lord, we pray for our friend, Lakshmi. God in Heaven, every student here . . ." Ida named each girl as she prayed, "needs you . . ." Before closing the prayer, she opened her eyes. "Does anyone else want to pray?"

A head nodded. "I want to try," one of the girls said. The sweet sound of her voice sounded like Lakshmi's.

Where is Lakshmi, Lord? She swallowed a lump in her throat.

Ida rose from her knees, and the girls followed her lead. She hoped the prayers calmed the girls the same way it calmed her.

"We'll begin our afternoon with reading." The girls opened their readers.

The afternoon dragged for Ida. She couldn't abandon the routine, but all she wanted to do was go to Lakshmi's house. Ida paced from one end of the room to the other, checking the girls' work, glancing out the open door, and trying to ignore the queasiness in her stomach. She couldn't wait any longer. Her calm was about to explode without knowing where Lakshmi was.

Ida stepped outside and motioned for Souri. The afternoon palm tree shadows covered the school yard. "Please go to Lakshmi's house to see if she has come home."

After a few minutes, the shuffling of feet caused Ida to stop teaching and open the door. Souri waited with news. Ida stepped outside and closed the door.

"No news of Lakshmi yet," he whispered. "Her father and several village men are searching for her."

Ida took a breath to compose herself. She couldn't allow the girls to walk home alone. Three hours since lunch and still no word of Lakshmi. Ida's heart sunk like the setting sun. "School's dismissed," Ida said.

The girls stacked their slates and readers on the bookshelf. Instead of the normal chatter, Ida didn't even hear a whisper. As usual the girls formed a circle around Ida.

To keep the routine normal, she prayed and read a Psalm, then said, "Souri and I will walk you home today. We'll walk all together until each one of you darlings is delivered to your home."

One girl raised her hand.

"Yes?" Ida nodded for her to speak.

"Missy Ammal, are you walking with us because Lakshmi didn't come back?"

Ida took a deep breath. If only the truth weren't so hard to speak sometimes. "Yes." She lowered her

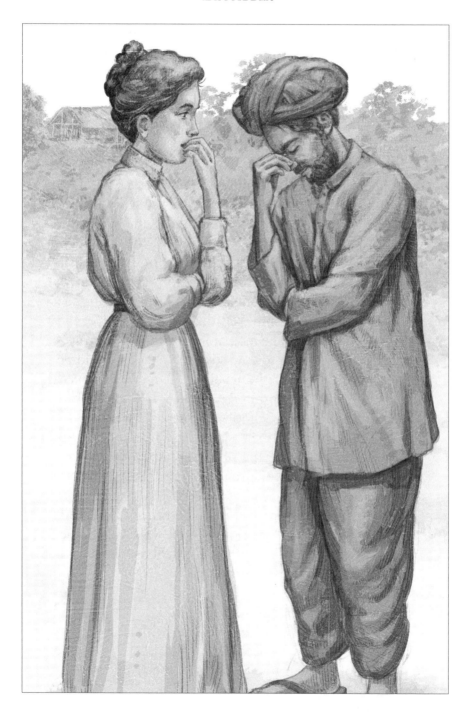

voice. She must say this gently. "Until I know Lakshmi is home, we'll walk together." She looked into each of their solemn eyes, hoping the calm in her face reassured them.

"Girls, we'll hook arms and walk as one big body as long as the path gives us enough room."

The students giggled and formed a line with Souri and then Mrs. Isaac on one end and Ida on the other.

CHAPTER 17

When Ida finished delivering each child to her home, she ran to the village. Inside Lakshmi's house, her mother sat in front of a small shrine with a clay statue, a tulsi plant, and a brass pot with burning incense.

"Have you found Lakshmi?" Ida said.

She shook her head. "We allowed her to learn about Christianity. The gods don't like what we did." The mother wiped a tear.

Ida knelt beside her. "A statue has no power—"

"Girls shouldn't go to school. The gods are punishing us for allowing Lakshmi to study like her brothers," the mother said, her voice weak and barely above a whisper.

"You mustn't think that." Ida wrapped an arm around the shoulders of Lakshmi's mother. "Educating a girl is the best thing to do for your daughter."

"If Lakshmi wasn't at school, she'd be home with me now." Tears streamed down her cheeks.

"I'll search the bazaar before it closes." Ida stood.

The mother nodded to acknowledge Ida but stayed planted on the ground in front of her shrine.

When Ida and Souri reached the mission, Souri prepared the pony cart to go to the bazaar. While they rode, Ida said, "I feel like I lost a daughter." Every minute made the sinking in her stomach worse. When Ida wasn't talking, she prayed in her mind. When they reached the busy bazaar, Ida searched the streets with Souri.

She rushed to the silver vendor first. How many times had Lakshmi played with her silver anklets and bracelets? The silver shop was empty except for the vendor sweeping the floor with a whisk broom. Ida's heart thumped. "Was there a school-age girl shopping this afternoon?"

"*Illia*. No schoolgirls here today."

Ida's hope plunged. She moved up the street searching and asking.

The vendors pulled the canvas over their shops. Ida didn't see Lakshmi anywhere. By sunset, Souri and Ida headed back to the bungalow. Ida dreaded the dark. How would they find Lakshmi at night?

The night ticked by slower than any night Ida had ever experienced. She couldn't sleep and finally gave up trying. Instead she prayed and read her Bible. The next morning she sent a mission worker to Lakshmi's house to find out if there was any news.

He returned a few minutes later, breathless from running. "No one has found Lakshmi."

All day Saturday Ida abandoned her chores to search for Lakshmi. By late afternoon she walked the path to the village, hoping and praying. Still Lakshmi wasn't home. Early Sunday morning Ida dressed for church and left to practice the hymns before service began. The routine didn't keep her mind off Lakshmi.

Although church didn't begin for another hour, Ida arrived to find villagers waiting at the door.

"Missy Ammal, did you hear?"

"Lakshmi? Did they find her?" Ida's heart leapt, hoping for good news.

A woman shook her head. "No. The parents received a postcard last night saying, 'You will find Lakshmi in a well.'"

Ida grabbed the doorjamb to steady herself. Resting her forehead against the wood, she allowed her tears to flow. After a few minutes, she composed herself and climbed on the organ bench. She went through the motions, but her mind wandered during the sermon. If only this moment weren't real. The minute church dismissed, Ida ran until she reached Lakshmi's house and found police officers talking with Lakshmi's father. She waited at the door.

One of the officers said, "We arrested three men who are responsible. They were looking for treasure and offered Lakshmi as a sacrifice for the goddess. They thought a child named after the goddess of prosperity would guarantee their success."

Ida covered her face with her hands. *Why, God?* She watched Lakshmi's father stiffen and his wife collapse in his arms.

Their home was already full of family and village neighbors who'd come to comfort the family. Seeing the family was comforted by so many, Ida slipped out to tell her parents.

When Ida arrived home, she found Marmee with Salomi preparing dinner. Ida told them the sad news.

Marmee took Ida's hand, guided her to the office, and patted the cushion on the settee.

Ida crumpled her body against her mother's and wept. A few minutes later, Ida dried her eyes with her sleeve. "September 9 is the worst day I've ever lived," Ida said.

"When we see evil at its worst," Marmee said, "we must remember who is behind it. Satan seeks whom he may devour."

"How will I face my students?" Ida blew her nose into a handkerchief.

Thunder rumbled outside. Rain pelted against the veranda. The pony cart pulled beside the bungalow, and Father ran through the rain to the office. He didn't hang his hat on the hook or set his medical bag on the desk. He walked straight to Ida and bent on the floor in front of her. "I heard. The news is all over Vellore."

Ida looked at her father's tender eyes. Her chin quivered and another spasm of tears flowed. "I'm heartbroken."

Marmee handed Ida a fresh handkerchief.

Father set his hat on the table and swiped a hand through his hair. "Remember the story of Cain and Abel in Genesis?"

"Yes."

"Man is capable of terrible evil outside of fellowship with God," Father said.

CHAPTER 18

Ida paced in the yard beside the classroom door on Tuesday morning. More than ever, she wanted to see the girls' lovely chestnut faces, hear their inquisitive voices, and watch their brown eyes alight when they learned something new. She needed a normal day as much as they needed one. But today must be different.

After Lakshmi's funeral, the village was quiet. Ida longed to hear the girls' laughter. Would her plans show the girls how to live in the safety of God and not in Satan's trap of fear? She said a silent prayer while she filled a bucket of water.

The ground was soggy from an overnight rain. Normally during monsoon season, Ida rinsed the girls' muddy feet with water. When she heard voices, she abandoned the empty bucket and ran up the path and greeted six girls. With each hug Ida's cheer resurrected like a spring flower after winter.

Ida walked back to the school with the first group. "Take a seat on your mat. I wrote the Bible verse on the chalkboard. Copy it in your best handwriting while I wait outside for the rest of the girls."

A few more arrived in pairs or walked together in small groups. One group arrived accompanied by a father. Ida waited fifteen minutes past normal starting time before she walked to the classroom. She sank to the floor beside the girls and counted—only a third of the class. "We're going to share all the ways Lakshmi made us smile."

A girl raised her hand. Her forehead was dotted with a red bindi between her eyes. "Lakshmi helped me up when I fell in the mud."

"She made faces to make me laugh," another girl said.

"Laughing is good medicine," Ida said.

"Lakshmi taught me how to jump rope," a girl said.

One by one the girls talked about Lakshmi. Their voices soothed Ida like water on a hot day. No matter how much she hurt or the girls hurt for the loss of Lakshmi, God would use time to soften their ache.

"I loved Lakshmi," a little girl said, whimpering.

Ida rubbed her back. "We all loved her, dearest." She opened her Bible. "I want to read to you what God says about love. In the book of Corinthians, chapter 13, it says, 'Charity suffereth long, and is kind.'" Ida looked up from her Bible. "Charity means love."

When no one responded, she continued, "'Is not easily provoked, thinketh no evil; Rejoiceth not in iniquity, but rejoiceth in the truth; Beareth all things, believeth all things, hopeth all things, endureth all things.'"

Ida studied the girls' faces to see if they understood. "Did you hear that love does not think evil?"

Several girls nodded.

"Iniquity means evil. God's love does not rejoice in evil. God is the opposite of evil. He is sad about Lakshmi too."

"I'm afraid," a girl in the front said.

"The men were arrested by the police. They are far away in a jail and can't hurt anyone again."

Surround my girls with your angels, Lord.

During the next six months, the village parents started sending their daughters back to school. By April, school attendance was nearly back to normal. Ida's heart ached since Lakshmi's death, but she'd found comfort reading her Bible. Her morning quiet time with God was more important than ever.

Each day Ida rose during the twilight of the morning hours, when the outdoors was still quiet, when she could be alone with Father. She combed her hair into a bun, slipped on a skirt and blouse, and shuffled to his office.

He sat at the desk chair with his Bible open.

"Good morning," Ida said, her voice a whisper.

Father's eyes peered over his glasses. "I knew you'd be here soon."

In mutual silence they both studied their Bibles before they spoke. For the past three years she cherished their morning routine. After thirty minutes of quiet, the birds chirped at the same time Father packed supplies in his worn medical bag.

Ida finished reading her Bible and wrote in her journal, noting her thoughts about patience. Father was a living example of God's patience and long-suffering. The more she watched him interact with his patients, the more she watched how he endured long work hours without complaint and his devotion to God, and the more she wanted to be like him.

Salomi delivered the morning chota at 6:00 a.m. The sounds of people taking their goats and wagons to market wafted through the open door. The silence between them broken, Father spoke. "I was thinking you ought to visit your cousin, Lew, in Ranipet. You'd get good exposure to patients in a hospital if you follow him on rounds."

Ida's heart thumped from the thought of being in a hospital among patients. "Didn't you start that hospital?" she asked.

Father nodded while he refilled medicine bottles from his doctor bag. "Yes, I converted old army barracks into a hospital when we lived in Ranipet. Then we moved to Vellore right after you were born. The hospital is primitive compared to hospitals in the US, but having a place to admit patients is important."

"I'd like to observe Lew, but I don't want to be a hindrance."

"How could anyone as bright as you be a hindrance? I want you to go into medicine with your eyes wide open. Cases in India won't be the same as the ones you'll treat in the US." Father winked at Ida.

Ida sipped the hot chota. "Do you think Vellore will ever have a hospital?"

"Vellore desperately needs a hospital." He closed his bag and shrugged into a suit jacket. "I'll write a letter to Lew to arrange your visit."

Two weeks later Ida boarded the train on a Friday morning and met Lew in Ranipet. Ida stepped off the train and moved through the crowd toward Lew.

"I'm going to put you to work right away." Lew led Ida to his pony wagon.

"Whatever I can do to assist, I will do," Ida said, tingling inside. "How about I take over the operations?" she laughed.

Within a few minutes, Lew parked in front of a cement building.

The stucco on it had peeled away in several places. Red sand stained the lower half of the building. The hospital wasn't anything like Ida imagined. Some of the windowpanes were missing. Even for an old army barrack, how could a hospital be inside such a ramshackle of a building?

Lew led Ida through a door. The wood on the door was splintered from sun and rain beating. They walked through the hospital ward, an open room with rows of beds on both sides of an aisle in the middle. Lew stopped at the first bed and told Ida about the patient.

Lew lifted the sheet. "I set this gentleman's broken leg."

Ida leaned over the patient for a closer look at the leg brace. He walked her past the patients, naming their diagnoses: dysentery, leprosy, malaria, Guinea worm.

A nurse ran to Lew. "Dr. Scudder, we have an emergency in the dispensary. A man was gored by a bull."

"Come on," Lew pulled Ida by the hand and followed the nurse into the dispensary at the opposite end of the hospital ward.

The patient moaned and writhed on the hospital bed.

"I've covered the wound with sterile cloths," the nurse said, "but the bleeding is impossible to stop."

Lew lifted the blood-soaked sheet. "This laceration isn't too deep." He let go of the sheet and scanned the room. "Ida, clean the area around the wound, and we'll stitch him back together."

Ida and Lew washed their hands and put on gloves. The nurse set out a tray of needles, gauze, and surgical thread.

The patient chewed on his knuckles and moaned. Tears seeped from the corner of his eyes.

Ida wiped his sweaty forehead with a wet washcloth. "You're going to feel better soon."

Lew bent over the patient, explaining as he worked. "I'd estimate this is a fifteen-inch wound across his buttocks. Lucky the bull didn't gore his abdomen, or it would have ruptured his organs."

Ida nodded, studying his skillful suturing.

Lew stopped and held the needle in the air. "Give it a try." He looked at Ida.

"Me? I shouldn't. I—"

"Why not? It's the perfect opportunity. You embroider, don't you?"

"Yes." Her heart thumped wildly. "But this isn't cloth."

Lew handed her the suture. "You finish the job. I'll supervise."

Ida's hand shook when she pushed the needle through the skin for the first time. She paused. This is what life will be like after medical school. She concentrated, trying to reproduce the exact stitches as Lew. Sweat covered her brow, but after a few times through the man's skin, she relaxed.

"Finished," Ida said at last, sighing. Her body ached from standing in one place. Being a doctor was going to take mental and physical stamina.

"Not bad for your first job," Lew said. "You'll learn."

CHAPTER 19

Ida returned from Ranipet wishing she could start medical school immediately, but she had another a year before she could leave. The next summer she arranged a graduation ceremony for the older girls at the church.

The evening of the graduation, the church filled with family and friends while the girls waited outside. Each girl wore her best sari. The line was a vivid display of color.

Ida stood back and surveyed the line, thinking over the past month of planning. Most of these girls, only eleven and twelve years old, would be married and carrying around their own children by the time she returned to Vellore.

One by one Ida called their names, and each girl came to the front. Marmee handed the diplomas out while Ida hugged each girl and whispered a personal compliment to each.

All the painstaking effort to plan this graduation was worth it. The moment was bittersweet for Ida—an ending for the girls and a beginning for her.

In August, Uncle Jared and his family returned to Vellore to switch places with Ida and her parents. Ida packed her belongings in the trunk she'd brought four years ago. When she emptied her desk, she found a small red diary where she had scribbled entries when she lived in the dorm at Northfield.

She flipped open a page dated January 1, 1890: "A very poor day for the beginning of the new year. I arrayed myself with a new green dress and started with Walter for a party. All my things look so badly. Wish I had lots of money."

Ida stared at the words. She wasn't the same person she was four years ago. She closed the diary, feeling a flush of embarrassment. Thank goodness God changed her heart. *I'm sorry, God, for not seeing how trivial my worries were compared to others.*

She tucked the diary into the bottom of the trunk, thinking of the Bible story of Lot's wife looking back. *Don't look back on your immaturity*, Ida chided herself. *You're twenty-four-years old and ready to face a new future.* She clicked the metal latches into place, patted the side of the wooden trunk, and spoke to it as if speaking to a friend—"See you in New York."

The next morning Ida, Marmee, and Father spent the day traveling to Madras. The waterfront city was busy with traffic from ships porting from around the world. Madras was modern with larger buildings in the downtown area. After a poor night's sleep in the noisy city, Ida and her parents boarded a ship to New York City.

Unlike the last voyage, Ida spent her mornings in quiet time. At the end of each day, she marked them off on a calendar with a giant X. She enjoyed the restful time playing shuffleboard with Father and board games with Marmee. Within two months Ida and her parents stood on the ship's deck along with hundreds of other passengers as they entered the New York harbor.

Moist air bathed Ida's face as the steamer passed through the morning fog. The torch on the Statue of Liberty came into view. The rest of the statue remained shrouded in mist. She clasped Marmee's hand in hers.

"India's thousands of miles behind us now," Marmee said.

"It's been a dream to come back for so long I can't believe I'm really here," Ida said, her heart pumping along with the frothy water.

As the steamer made headway through the harbor, the sun burned off the fog. The statue came into full view.

"She's magnificent," Father said. "I've seen magazine photos of the statue, but the real view is—"

"Beautiful, and somehow, overwhelming." Ida shut her eyes. The impact of the moment solidified her decision. There was no turning back now.

"You're like the Lady of Liberty for India, holding a torch for the women of Vellore," Marmee said.

Father pulled a brochure out of his front coat pocket and read, " 'The statue means *Liberty Enlightening the World*.' "

"That's our Ida," Marmee said. "She's lighting the way."

New York's tall buildings lined the horizon. Seagulls dipped in and out of the harbor. A few passengers tossed chunks of bread into the air for the gulls. One caught a chunk in midair.

"I have a massive amount of work to do first," Ida said, feeling like a gull trying to find a piece of bread on the ocean's surface. "Will I accomplish all the tasks in front of me?"

"With God, for He is all powerful," Marmee said.

"Yes, and He's capable of helping you accomplish what He's sent you to do." Father winked.

Ida took a deep breath. "Yes, *with God all things are possible.*"

Before leaving New York City, Ida and her parents visited old friends, Katherine Van Nest and Myra Moffat, at West 56th Street.

After a supper of roast beef, Katherine asked their housekeeper to bring tea to the sitting room. Myra led them near the front entrance to an ornate sitting room with wallpapered walls and dark, mahogany furniture.

Father and Marmee sat together on another settee on the opposite side of the room.

Katherine helped the housekeeper serve. "How long are you visiting the States?" Myra said.

"Our sons, Walter and Henry, are enrolled in seminary." Marmee sipped her cup tea.

"We're going to live with them in New Brunswick, New Jersey, for our two-year furlough," Father said.

Ida stirred the hot tea, sloshing it onto the saucer. What was she going to do about tuition? Seminary must be cheaper than medical school. Asking the mission board to support a missionary going to seminary was logical. How was she going to convince them to support medical school for a woman?

"When do you start school?" Myra said, interrupting Ida's thoughts.

"The Women's Medical College accepted my application on the condition I take the Regent's Exam." Her stomach knotted up with the conversation. She scooted to the edge of her chair, her back rigid. "I have a few months to study before the exam later this fall. If I pass, I'll begin school in January."

"Where are you going to stay?" Katherine said.

"I'll find a hostel or the YWCA," Ida said.

"Stay with us," Myra said, adjusting in her chair.

"What belongs to us is yours." Katherine nodded.

"If you need to go to the library to study, our carriage driver will take you," Myra said.

"I appreciate the offer," Ida beamed, "which I accept. I didn't relish the idea of lodging in a strange place."

A week later Ida traveled to the train station to see her parents off for New Brunswick.

"I'll miss you," Ida said.

Marmee tucked a stray hair behind Ida's ear like she used to do when Ida was a girl. "You'll join us in New Brunswick after your exam, yes?"

Ida nodded, wondering why she was trembling. She was one step closer to school. One step closer to the center of God's will. Would she achieve her plans?

Father kissed Ida's forehead. "You're going to be a wonderful doctor."

Ida closed her eyes. "I'm feeling fragile right now," she whispered.

As the conductor called for passengers, Ida pecked her parents' cheeks. They boarded and waved good-bye from their window seat.

For a moment Ida's mind flashed back to her boarding school years as a girl living away from her parents. As the reality of starting medical school settled in, apprehension filled her. She'd prayed and waited and dreamt of this adventure. Why did she feel like a bird being pushed out of its nest, even though she wanted wings to fly?

CHAPTER 20

Ida spent the winter researching in books, jotting notes in her journal, and reviewing. Early on a Monday morning, four months since she'd arrived in New York, Ida rode a carriage to the City University for the Regent's Exam. On the way Ida flipped through the review cards she'd made to quiz herself, but her mind raced past the words.

She put the cards into her purse, took a deep breath, and instead, repeated the Bible verse she'd memorized. "'And the peace of God, which passeth all understanding, shall keep your hearts and minds through Christ Jesus.' Philippians 4:7."

When Ida reached the four-story brick building, her stomach roiled. Four years was a long time to be out of school. If she didn't pass this test, she'd never make it into medical school.

Up a flight of steps Ida found the correct classroom filled with a roomful of people waiting silently for the test. A chalkboard covered the wall behind a teacher's desk. Rows of desks filled the remainder of the classroom.

She slipped into an empty desk in the front row. A teacher stood beside the desk, holding his pocket watch in his hand.

Ida put her hand against her stomach. A flock of butterflies fluttered inside. She tapped the eraser end of her pencil on the desk.

At precisely 9:00 a.m., the instructor cleared his throat, picked up the exams, and spoke. "Directions are on the board, but I will read them to you anyway." He half-turned and read the directions in a monotone voice. When finished, he faced the classroom. "Any questions?"

No one raised their hand.

"Fine. When you're finished, turn your test booklet over and remain in your seat until the exam ends. I will call time every hour for a five-minute bathroom break."

At the two-hour bathroom break, Ida was excited, even though her brain was tired. She thought she was doing well. Thirty minutes later, Ida double-checked her answers and turned over her exam. At noon, the instructor collected the exams from everyone. Ida glided through the hallway, across the wooden floor, and down the concrete step to the waiting carriage.

When she returned to 56th Street, Katherine and Myra stood in the foyer awaiting her arrival. "Time to celebrate. Your test is over." Myra adjusted her hat.

Katherine opened the door, and at the carriage told the driver. "We're off for a soda." Fifteen minutes later the driver parked in front of a pharmacy.

Ida helped Myra climb onto a stool in front of the soda fountain, before she sat between her house hosts.

Wearing a white uniform, a pharmacist held a pen and paper in his hand. "What can I get you ladies?"

"We'll have three cream sodas, please," Katherine said.

Ida grinned. "You two are such fun. Thank you for your hospitality."

"We've adored your company," Katherine said.

"You make us feel youthful." Myra sipped the soda with a straw.

"About tomorrow," Katherine said. "Are you ready to speak to the women's board at 9:00 a.m.?"

Ida nodded and sipped her soda.

"After the meeting we'll whisk you to the train station for New Brunswick to see your parents," Myra said.

The next morning, Ida selected her mission outfit, a long dark skirt and high-necked, white blouse. Fashion wasn't a priority at the moment, even though a new outfit for speaking would have been nice. When they arrived at Collegiate Church, a white-marbled structure, Ida took deep breaths to calm her pounding heart as she walked past the high-columned entrance.

Ida peeked inside the sanctuary. A large pipe organ flanked the front wall beside the arched ceiling. The ornate room was a stark contrast to the mud-hut churches in India. A lady with a bucket scrubbed the wooden banisters. Inside, the building smelled like lemon furniture oil.

"The sanctuary is breathtaking," Ida whispered.

Katherine led the way to a Sunday school room for the meeting and held the door open. Against the wall where they entered, a table covered with a white cloth displayed cookies, tea, and coffee. Ida placed a cookie on her plate to be polite, but none of the treats appealed to her. She just wanted her talk to be done.

Ida picked at the handkerchief she'd hid beneath the cuff on her blouse and watched the room full of women, wondering if they would be receptive to her. The women wore stylish hats covered in feathers, flowers, or giant bows in purples, greens, and browns. Their perfume filtered through the air as they talked to one another. Myra and Katherine mingled with friends and introduced Ida, then led her to the chairs lined in front near the podium.

Ten minutes later a minister walked to the podium and opened the meeting with prayer. After the secretary read the minutes from the last meeting and the treasurer reported, the missionary auxiliary president introduced Ida. "As members of the mission board, you know the long history of Scudder missionaries in India. Today I'd like to introduce you to a member of the family, Miss Ida Scudder. She is home from a four-year term in India and will share a few experiences with us today."

The saliva in Ida's mouth dried like someone had swiped her tongue with a sock. *Dear Lord, please speak for me.* She cleared her throat and approached the podium.

From behind the podium, Ida looked at the faces staring back at her. "Imagine living behind the walls of a courtyard since birth. You are twelve years old, and your only companions are your mother, grandmother, aunts, and cousins. On your wedding day from behind your bridal veil, you might glimpse a view of the city you've never seen. A curtained cart will take you to live in a new zenana with your husband."

"Child marriage is not illegal in India. Girls become mothers by age fourteen or younger. According to the Hindu and Muslim laws, only a man in the immediate family may see their wives and children. There isn't

117

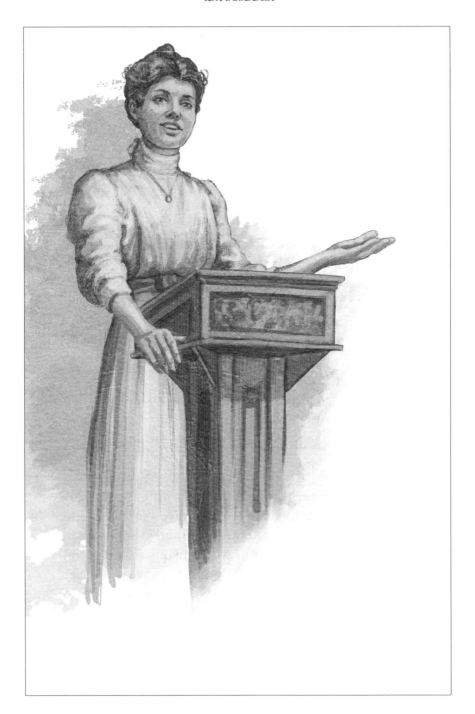

a female doctor for the women to treat preventable deaths.

"Two years ago, during a single night, three different husbands came to me." Ida's voice broke. She wiped her eyes and took a deep breath. "Each husband needed a woman doctor to save his wife." Ida repeated the story of that pivotal night. "By dawn when I heard the death song of the tom-tom, I knew what God wanted me to do with my life. I stayed on my knees and prayed. God showed me I could be a doctor for these women. That morning I promised God I would serve the women in India. Thank you for allowing me to share my story."

Her neck and cheeks burned. Grateful she was finished, Ida took her seat. Myra patted her knee and mouthed, "Good job, dear."

The president walked to the podium. "Ida, we appreciate your sincerity. You told an emotional story that, I can say, has profoundly affected me." She paused. "Now Miss Kate Van Nest has a few remarks."

Katherine stood and walked to the podium. "Thank you, Ida." She grinned as she looked directly at Ida.

"As you heard, Ida is committed to life as a missionary doctor." Katherine looked out at the audience. "She hopes to enroll at the Women's Medical College in Pennsylvania. Ida will live with her parents in New Brunswick until the next semester begins in January. Although our bylaws don't permit us to pay for her tuition, I do know we could present personal gifts to her. I suggest we send this young lady to medical school so she can fulfill her promise to God and her promise to the women she left behind in Vellore. The tuition for one year is $141.50. Thank you."

Katherine returned to her chair, and the president walked to the podium. "We're open for discussion," she said.

For a moment, no one spoke up. The silence stretched on until it became awkward. Ida looked down and prayed that someone would speak soon.

A woman wearing a moss green outfit and feather hat spoke first. Ida looked in that direction. "Society, even in America, is distrustful of the few women doctors in our country," she said. "After what you've shared, how would India accept a female doctor?"

Myra spoke. "My understanding is the majority work in other countries as missionaries."

Katherine knocked on the podium. "The medical school in Pennsylvania opened over forty years ago. We must celebrate progress."

"The expenditure is a waste," a woman wearing a hat with a giant flower said. "No one will believe in a woman as a competent doctor."

A few hats bobbed in agreement.

Another woman wearing all black spoke. "It's not even proper to send an unmarried lady doctor to the mission field."

Ida's heart skipped a beat. She turned in time to see Myra scowl.

People rustled in their seats, coughed, cleared their throats, but no one stood to support Ida.

Ida took her handkerchief and wiped her nose. She wanted to cover her face, but Myra pulled her hand into hers.

"Stay strong, dear," Myra whispered.

I don't have anywhere else to turn. Is this the end of my dream, God?

CHAPTER 21

Ida wondered how it was possible for her to cry and laugh at the same time, until she looked at Katherine.

Back at the apartment in the sitting room, Ida, Katherine, and Myra discussed the morning event at Collegiate. Katherine slung herself onto the settee. Myra followed Katherine's lead, landing with a thump on the brocade chair. Myra covered her mouth and tittered and rung the bell for their housekeeper.

Unable to squelch her excitement, Ida walked in a circle, holding the sides of her head. "I can't believe it."

"Your face is all a'flush," Myra said. "A perfect match to the brocade chair cushion."

Ida sat on the tip of the needlepoint chair. "I'm speechless."

"No wonder, after a morning like we had." Katherine held her head against the back of the settee.

The housekeeper walked in and set a silver tea set on the marble serving table. The sunlight from the window reflected a prism of color from the crystal sugar dish, matching the spirit in the room. Talking at the same time, Ida, Katherine, and Myra each told different aspects of the morning.

"My gracious. Slow down. I can't understand any of you," the housekeeper said.

Myra patted the settee. "Sit with us a moment before we start lunch. We have a wonderful story to tell."

"We're delirious with joy." Katherine stood. "After several of the ladies protested the idea of Ida going to medical school, the room turned as silent as a tomb." She paused and acted as if she were on a stage. "But then, a lovely young lady stood—"

"The one wearing a purple hat," Ida said.

"And she waved her money," Myra said.

Katherine mimicked the lady in the purple hat. "I support Miss Ida Scudder's decision to attend medical school, and here is the first ten dollars toward the tuition."

"Then another lady stood and pledged her money," Myra said.

"The one with the moss green hat." Ida leaned forward. "The morning started out poorly. Then everything reversed. I hardly believe it really happened."

"God creates miraculous situations, doesn't He?" Myra said.

The housekeeper dropped sugar cubes in each cup and passed them out.

"And one right after the other dropped a contribution into the basket," Katherine said.

"Until we had exactly $141.50." Katherine stretched out her arms.

The housekeeper set the last teacup beside Ida and covered her mouth. "Oh my!"

Myra started to sing. "Praise God from whom all blessings flow."

Katherine and Ida finished singing the hymn with her.

The next morning Ida looked around at the stylish apartment. She stood beside the door in the foyer, a purse wrapped around her shoulder and a suitcase on the floor beside her. Katherine and Myra stood on either side of Ida.

"You are both so kind and generous," Ida said. "I feel like family."

"Think of me as a doting aunt," Myra said.

"Consider me your big sister," Katherine said.

"I wouldn't be able to enter medical school this fall if it hadn't been for your guidance. I sincerely appreciate both of you." Ida hugged Kate and then Myra. "You've been a blessing to me. I love you both dearly."

Ida stepped outside where dogwood blossoms covered the ground. She paused to take in the vibrant green of the trees covered in dew before she bounced down the steps, climbed into the carriage, and blew a kiss to her "doting aunt" and "big sis" watching from the stoop. She felt like a princess being whisked away from the ball, with yet another ball—medical school—to attend.

At the train station Ida settled in with her journal for the hour ride. The short ride between New York and New Brunswick was just enough time to think through the past few weeks and collect her thoughts. When the train conductor opened the doors, Ida bounced off the train, spotted Father and Marmee, and ran to them.

"You have good news, don't you?" Marmee said. "I can tell by the way your eyes sparkle."

Ida squeezed Marmee and Father in a hug like a lost child who'd found her parents. "God is so good to me." She focused on Father's eyes. "You were right. God provided the tuition for my first year in medical school."

Three weeks later after arriving in New Brunswick and staying with her parents at the parsonage, Ida's Regent Exam scores arrived, along with a letter of congratulations from the Medical College for Women in Pennsylvania.

Ida scanned the typed letter, running her hands over the school's name embossed at the top and at the bottom with the dean's signature, Dr. Clara Marshall, WMCP. The letter. A symbol of approval. Another opened door from God.

"I passed."

"Of course, you did," Marmee said.

She exhaled a heavy breath. "I'm officially enrolled in medical school for the 1895 school year." Ida tapped her lip with her finger. "In 1899, I'll be Dr. Ida Scudder."

In January, Father and Marmee traveled with Ida to Philadelphia. After the train trip, they took a carriage to Arch Street. When they arrived, Ida ran her hand across the embossed wooden sign and read it aloud, "The Women's College of Medicine in Pennsylvania."

Father and Marmee toured the three-story red brick school with Ida. They spent time in each classroom. "The building reminds me of the architecture at Northfield," Ida said.

Inside, Ida lingered in the anatomy and physiology classroom, studying the body charts and the skeleton.

"Wish I could take a class," Father said.

An hour later Ida and her parents walked to the students' residence down the street from the school. Ida and her parents spent time in the sitting room of the residence and met several other ladies enrolled in medical school. With each introduction, Ida knew she was in the right place.

After a brief visit with the other students, Ida walked her parents to the porch to tell them goodbye.

"One last hug," Marmee said. "Remember, if you need us, we are only a hundred miles away, not halfway around the globe. I missed so much of your teen years. I don't ever want to miss that much time with you again."

"Me either." Ida laughed, remembering her immature teenage pranks.

"No pranks." Father chuckled. "I don't want any letters from the dean."

"Absolutely." Ida winked at Father and waved goodbye.

———

That night Ida met her roommates, Sylvia, Margaret, and Nell, all first-year medical students, and the next day the four of them waited forty-five-minutes in line to register for classes.

When Ida reached the table, the registrar handed Ida her schedule. "Five days a week of class from nine to five and clinical with the doctors at the Pennsylvania Doctors' Hospital every Saturday morning."

Ida lugged the thick books back to her room. The next morning classes began. Ida's day began with chemistry, followed by a lab, therapeutic class, and then surgery observations all afternoon in the operating theater.

Each day was different with classes in dermatology to obstetrics to dental surgery. She raced to keep up with notes. During surgery, she sketched the details of everything she watched. In the evenings, she studied with her roommates. On Saturdays the medical students practiced alongside doctors during clinics at the Pennsylvania Hospital.

"I'm already bleary-eyed," Ida said to her roommates at the end of the first week. "Now I wish Northfield had offered more chemistry classes. I have more background knowledge in literature than organic chemistry."

"I heard the Eta Chi Sorority offers their members tutoring and group study sessions," Nell said.

"Tutoring in chemistry?" Ida said. "I'm joining."

Ida loved making friends with the other medical students at Eta Chi. Each student took their classes seriously, and the study sessions improved grades. After receiving her grades, she wrote home.

Dear Father and Marmee,

So far school's going well, but I've struggled with chemistry. I've worried endlessly about my scores, but I'm happy to report I made an A on my first chemistry test. How I wish I could celebrate with you. See you at Christmas.

Your loving daughter, Ida

Before Christmas, one of Ida's classmates from Eta Chi developed a fever and a cough.

"Did you hear they're sending Louise home?" Nell said.

"Why?" Ida's body tensed.

"She caught tuberculosis," Margaret said.

Ida's pulse skipped a beat. Losing a classmate to tuberculosis worried her. "I can't bear the thought of Louise dealing with a terminal disease. She didn't even make it to Christmas."

"We're working under pressure—rigorous classes, demanding schedule, lack of sleep, plus exposure to germs during our clinical time at the hospital," Nell said. "I'm not surprised Louise turned sick."

"I feel so bad for her," Ida said. She looked off in the distance through the bedroom window, feeling weak and exposed. *Dear God, if I end up sick, how will I ever help the women in India?*

CHAPTER 22

Ida and the close-knit group of the Eta Chi students bonded like drops of water attaching to one another. She discovered everyone faced the same fear of catching a disease from their patients. Ida and her roommates formed an even tighter inner circle, doctoring each other by giving "prescriptions of bed rest," for anyone who looked pale, peaked, or strained. They reminded each other to "scrub your hands," after hospital rounds.

Neither Ida nor her roommates caught anything beyond a head cold, but two of the girls, Jeannette and Rachel from Eta Chi, caught typhoid fever soon after the winter term began. Ida's heart ached for her sick classmates. Back in her room one night after a long day of classes, she rummaged around for a rag and went into a cleaning frenzy.

"It's hard to accept how out of control we really are," Ida said, dusting the top of her desk.

"Satan is going to try and throw us off course," Nell said. "We have to rely on prayer."

"And use the good sense God gave us," Sylvia said.

"And maybe, limit our cleaning to once a week?" Margaret held Ida's histology textbook toward her. "We have a lab exam tomorrow."

Ida tossed the dirty rag into the laundry basket, accepted the book, and opened it to the bookmarked page. "Back to the books," she said, plopping onto her bed.

With time, Ida relaxed into the school routine and stopped fretting over catching a disease. Time passed swiftly. With six days of classes and clinics, she didn't even have time for a prank.

On Saturdays, clinicals at the hospital included an hour for the medical students to question the doctors after patient exams were over. One day after treating patients with the supervising doctors, the medical students and two doctors met in the doctor's lounge at the hospital. Softened leather chairs and worn sofas bordered the walls. A coffee table, occupying the middle of the room, was covered with medical reference books. Two windows on the outer wall overlooked downtown Philadelphia.

Ida and a dozen fellow students packed themselves into the chairs and sofas. After the follow-up of each patient's diagnosis with a female physician, a male Indian doctor opened the discussion. "Any discussion or questions?"

Ida's mind often pondered the problems she'd encounter in India. "I've read about the new cholera vaccine. In India they don't accept anything with animal products. The stabilizer is made with ghee, which provides a safe vaccine for those opposed to animal tissue."

"A vaccine that can knock out cholera will save thousands of lives." The doctor cleared his throat. "Since I'm from India, I think I can speak with authority. The vaccine isn't the answer to the problem. Without doubt, your biggest hurdle will be convincing the Indian people to accept a shot."

"Yes," Ida scooted deeper in her seat, "I've heard of the struggles. My father is a doctor in southern India. He wrote to me that he took the vaccine in front of a group of villagers so they wouldn't be afraid of it."

The female doctor chimed in. "I'll give you another hurdle to conquer. Forget working in India or even in America."

A murmur traveled through the room. Suddenly the plain surroundings felt cold and austere like a gray sky. Ida bristled. *Who is she to tell me I can't do something? I'll prove her wrong.* Ida glanced at Nell, whose pinched expression told her they were both annoyed.

"Being accepted as a female doctor, even in America, is one obstacle after another. I'd advise you to cut your hair, wear a suit, and pretend to be a man." The doctor crossed her arms. "Your life will be much easier."

A wave rippled up Ida's spine. Ida scooted to the edge of her chair. How could a female doctor working with female medical students advise them to retreat?

The doctor ran her hands through her hair. "Go to Paris to work where they accept females as physicians. I'm leaving in December."

Ida felt the heat rise up her neck.

"I must disagree," the Indian doctor said. "The Women's Medical College opened forty-five years ago, and the number of graduates increases every year."

Nell spoke and looked at the female doctor. "You have my respect, doctor. But," she turned toward Ida, "you must realize we didn't choose medicine because it was going to be easy." She looked around the room at her classmates. Many nodded.

"I think Nell speaks for the majority of women in this room," Ida said. "We don't plan to run from trouble."

Several students answered with an audible, "Yes."

"Fine debate, ladies," the Indian doctor said. "Let's adjourn." He stood and opened the door.

After the meeting at the hospital, Ida talked with her classmates in the sitting room of the residence hall. "I suppose the doctor wanted to discourage us. For me, her comments only fueled my determination."

By February, winter snow laced the streets in bundles of white. Ida had loved the winter weather ever since her growing up days. The temperatures hovered below freezing for most of February. Before the sun thawed the snow into soupy puddles and mudpie streets, another snowstorm swept the earth white again.

Each day, she lifted her dress to keep it from gathering snow at the hem and prayed silently on her walk to classes, thanking God for protecting her from sickness.

By April, Ida beamed at the new sprouts of green earth and blooms in the trees. She continued studying like a soldier on duty, rising before the sun to review and rewrite her notes until she'd memorized everything. Even after Saturday clinics, she'd visit the library to read medical texts.

After the end of the school year, Ida worked in the hospital for the summer. For a one-week vacation, she met her parents and brothers in New Brunswick.

The tips of the maple-tree leaves were tinged in reds and yellows when Ida returned for the second year of medical school. She bounced down the sidewalk, feeling more confident than the previous year. She knew the professors, knew her roommates, and knew a little bit about medicine.

At the first Eta Chi study group meeting that fall, she rejoiced to see the membership swell with new medical students. Her former classmates, Rachel and Jeannette, re-enrolled as first-year medical students after their battle with typhoid.

On the weekends whenever possible, Ida and her friends hiked to East Fairmount Park and around the reservoir, a man-made lake built as a source of drinking water. At the park the girls met male students from the University of Pennsylvania Medical School. Students from both schools socialized together on the weekends at either the men's or women's residence parlor. Ida looked forward to the taffy pulling, chess matches, and charades.

Occasionally Ida accepted an invitation from one of the men to attend church, a concert, or challenge one another in a tennis match.

In the privacy of their room, Nell teased Ida. "You receive so many social invitations from the men, you might be a Dr. and Dr. duo someday." Nell fiddled with her ring finger.

"My mind's too occupied to think of romance right now," Ida said, although the question lingered in her mind. Would she meet a husband before she left for India? She shook her head. *I can't consider that.* As usual Ida launched herself into studies like a starved man eating a meal.

The next summer arrived faster than Ida thought possible. She met her parents in New Brunswick, traveled to Long Island, and took a ferry to Shelter Island. Ida's entire family met for a reunion, including her brother John with his wife and children from California, and brother Lewis and his wife and children from the Nebraska farm. She hadn't seen them in two years since her return from India.

The summer was filled with tennis matches, boat trips, clambakes, and evening fireside sing-a-longs with her family.

One night beside a fire on the beach, Ida roasted an ear of corn. "I think my face might crack from smiling and laughing," Ida said.

"I hear your cousin Lewis sent for another doctor to work with him in Ranipet," Father said. "A newly graduated medical student named Louisa Hart."

"Two more years and I'll be in India," Ida said. How her heart longed to be there. "I wish I could go right now. I can almost smell the spices."

At the end of the summer of 1897, Father and Marmee prepared to return to Vellore. Ida told them goodbye before she returned to Philadelphia for her junior year. "I feel like an incomplete puzzle and the last piece doesn't fit until we're reunited."

CHAPTER 23

The summer of sunshine and water had invigorated Ida. Even though she missed her parents, she focused on classes and tamped down any loneliness. Dealing with the distance between them was far easier now that she was an adult.

By the weekend Ida's feet ached from standing for hours during labs, her hands hurt from note taking during lectures, and her eyes needed a rest from the strain of reading into the late-night hours. But now halfway through her third year of school, she was getting accustomed to the physical strain of medical work. For Christmas, after a brief visit with Katherine and Myra in New York, she worked at the Philadelphia Hospital.

The morning of January 2, 1898, Ida poured herself a cup of coffee. Upstairs a couple of girls slept, including her roommate, Nell. The remainder of her class chums should return from their visits home later in the day.

With an hour to spare before she reported to the hospital for work, she settled in an armchair at the dining room table to read the newspaper. A short column at the bottom of the inside page caught her attention. Ida stood and raced up the stairs to wake Nell, but stopped just before she turned the door handle. Nell worked the night shift at the hospital. She deserved to sleep.

The Eta Chi meeting was the time to show everyone the article. Ida gathered her coat, gloves, and hat from the clothes tree in the foyer, stuffed the newspaper into her coat pocket, and left on foot for the hospital, whistling all the way.

———

By seven o'clock that evening, the residence was a buzz of friends catching up with one another. A golden glow from the gas pendant lights and the fireplace lit the room. Around the parlor, the girls packed the room tight as a bird's nest. Some had to sit on the floor or lean against the wall, their long brown and black dresses contrasted against the light-blue wallpaper.

Five minutes later the meeting began. "Welcome back." Rosalee, the Eta Chi president, smiled. After a few announcements, she opened the discussion. "Does anyone have any matters we need to discuss before we end the business meeting?"

Ida raised her hand.

Rosalee nodded in Ida's direction. "Miss Scudder?"

"I'd like to read a newspaper article to the group." Ida unfolded the crinkled paper.

"I know what you're going to read," blurted a medical student. "The Cornell announcement."

"Yes." Ida grinned. "'Cornell Medical College Receives Endowment and Opens Door to Admit Women.'" She read the short article, watching the surprised faces as she shared the Cornell invitation. The announcement hung in the air for a second, then the room erupted in applause. Ida took her seat beside Nell.

"Cornell? Imagine graduating from such a prestigious university," a student said.

"I think we stay together at WMCP to show the men we don't need them." The medical student who'd interrupted Ida earlier crossed her arms.

"We're on equal ground with men now," Nell said. "That's progress."

"The article said Cornell Medical School is accepting women due to the endowment," another student said. "Not because they believe women can learn as well as men."

Another student rubbed her hands against her skirt. "My father would never allow me to attend classes with men."

"Sounds like we're an experiment. The women of WMCP ought to band together and boycott Cornell."

"Even if we were accepted," another student said, "would transferring our classes put us behind?"

Ida enjoyed listening to the different opinions.

"I suggest we end the business portion of our meeting and proceed to celebrate the new year," Rosalee said. She waved her hand over the lace-covered table in the middle of the room laden with an array of pears, apples, dates, figs, almonds, Brazil nuts, and homemade ginger cookies.

Ida and Nell followed the line around the table until their plates were covered with a sample of everything.

"Only sixteen more months and we'll graduate." Nell scooped a cup of mulled apple cider.

Ida led Nell to the foyer. "I've been wanting to talk with you since this morning," Ida said in an excited whisper. "What do you think about Cornell?"

"I'm interested. The teaching hospital for WMCP isn't as large as it should be," Nell said.

"New York could offer more clinical experiences than we'd encounter here," Ida said. Her heart thumped wildly every time she thought about Cornell. A bigger school and classes with male students sounded exciting.

Around the parlor the other women stood in pockets of three to four. A low murmur of conversations echoed throughout the room. Ida wondered if anyone was discussing Cornell. Ida and Nell circulated the room along with their roommates, Margaret and Sylvia.

The clock on the mantel chimed eight o'clock. Nell gathered the empty plates from the people around her. Ida and her roommates cleared the parlor table of food and washed the dishes before they went to their room. Back in the room, Margaret and Sylvia unpacked. Tired from a full day, Ida opened her bureau drawer and pulled out a nightgown.

"What if Cornell changes their mind?" Margaret said. "And you lose your slot here?"

"Are you thinking about transferring to Cornell?" Sylvia said, removing clothes and toiletries from her suitcase.

"I'm not missing an opportunity like this." Nell scooted onto the double bed.

Sylvia slid her suitcase under the bed. "I'll need to consult my family first."

Ida stared at the delicate rose wallpaper for a few seconds. "Father would support this idea, I'm sure." She looked at her Bible sitting on the nightstand beside her bed. "If I've learned anything so far, it's that God is in charge of my journey. I'll need to pray about this decision."

The next week Ida, Nell, Margaret, and Sylvia attended classes and studied like worker ants. When the four gathered in their room in the evening, no matter how late, they knelt together to pray. Ida wrote her parents, asking for advice and prayer. Each day that passed, she was more resolved to apply to Cornell.

CHAPTER 24

1898

Three months passed. The calendar read April. The dogwoods promised to bloom any day now, but the mail wasn't producing any letters from Cornell. Ida, Nell, Margaret, and Sylvia had lifted the squeaky letter box outside the front door several times a day over the past few weeks.

Mid-April, Ida arrived home to eat lunch before bacteriology lab started. Four white envelopes tucked inside the letter box waited like little hatchlings in a nest. Ida checked the names and found one addressed to her. The noon sun warmed the porch, and Ida stood in its rays to read the letter. From a distance, the bells from the Church of the Holy Trinity chimed the twelve o'clock hour.

Ripping the envelope, she stared at the first line as if it were alive—*Congratulations*. Ida mumbled as she read through the letter as if at a speed-reading contest. The next word her eyes paused on—*Accepted*.

Ida clapped her hands together. She wanted to parade on the street and do a jig. Or stand on a rooftop

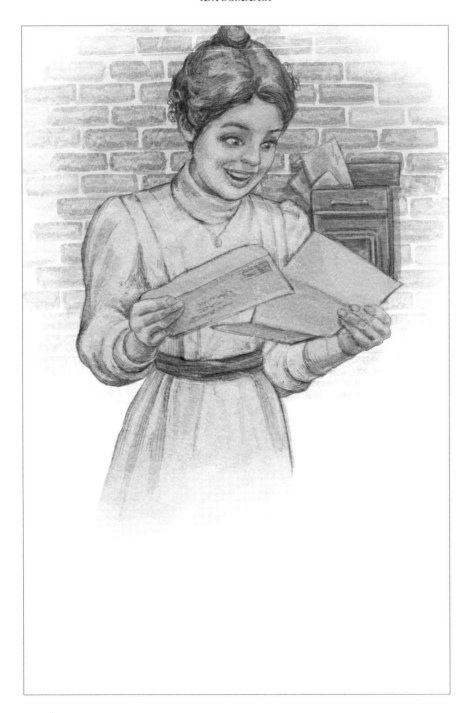

and shout to the people bustling by on the sidewalk—
Hey, did you know I was accepted to Cornell?

Instead of hand-delivering the other letters, she
slid the mail back into the letter box. The girls could
discover the surprise themselves. A pang shot through
Ida's chest. She'd have to hold back her enthusiasm in
case any of the others weren't accepted.

Hastily, Ida hid her acceptance letter inside a book.

That night in their room her roommates opened
their acceptance letters. "Everyone is going to
Cornell," Ida said.

"It's such good news," Nell said.

Sylvia did a mini-jump, and Margaret trotted
around the room embracing everyone. The four talked
at once. A thump on the door silenced them.

Ida opened the door.

Rosalee stood with her hands folded in front of her.

"Were we too loud?" Ida said.

Rosalee smiled. "I heard a lot of laughter."

Ida grabbed her hand and pulled her in the room.
"We're going to Cornell."

"I'm thrilled for you." Rosalee grinned. "I consid-
ered Cornell, but my father didn't approve. He said,
'Male and female students studying together is not
suitable for my daughter.'"

"I'm sorry." Margaret frowned.

"Convincing him to send me to medical school
was hard enough. At least I'm studying medicine."
Rosalee took a deep breath and smacked her hands
on her thighs. Her dress billowed at the hem. "Eta Chi
will plan a taffy pull and invite the men medical students to celebrate with you."

By the end of the month, Ida's summer plans were
made. In a letter from Katherine and Myra, they
begged her to live with them.

In early May, a letter from her parents arrived to confirm their approval of Cornell. Ida tingled all over. Every piece of the puzzle of her life was fitting together.

The weekend before the spring semester ended, the Eta Chi Sorority hosted the goodbye taffy pull for Ida, Nell, Sylvia, and Margaret. The men arrived as Rosalee poured the hot sugar mixture into a large, buttered pan to cool. The kitchen smelled sweet like a bakery.

By summer, Ida found herself caught up in paper-work. She visited New Brunswick and rushed to have every form completed and school credits transferred to Cornell. She wrote to Annie Hancock to update her and confirmed their visit to Northfield later in the summer. By late-summer, her brother Charles married Millie. After the wedding, Ida spent the last few days visiting with Walter before she moved to New York.

On the first morning of Ida's visit at the parsonage in New Brunswick, Walter prepared breakfast. "Sis, you looked beautiful in your bridesmaid's dress. And your roommate, Nell Bartholomew, looked like an angel. Where have you been hiding her?"

"You've met Nell before." Ida winked at Walter. "She's attending Cornell, and you'll only be an hour away. Come for a visit."

He grinned.

Two days later Ida took the train to New York. Myra's and Katherine's carriage driver met her at the train station. When she arrived at West 56th Street, Ida noticed movement behind the window. Myra and Katherine stood at the window and waved.

Ida climbed out of the carriage. By the time she was on the sidewalk, Katherine and Myra swung the apartment door open and stepped out on the stoop.

"Our girl is here," Myra said.

Ida held her skirt up and bounded toward them. Her heart was full, as if she were visiting family. "Let me hug you." She smiled and looked up at the familiar stone on the apartment. "I'm home."

———————

A week later, Ida arrived at Cornell. With the East River flowing on one side, the Cornell campus boasted several administration buildings on the roomy campus. Ida opened the double door of the Cornell Administration Building to meet Nell, Sylvia, and Margaret, who stood inside not far from the doorway.

Ida beamed at her friends. "Frankly, I'm shaking," she said under her breath.

"I'm glad we decided on this meeting," Margaret said. "A seven-hundred-acre campus is much larger than WMCP."

Sylvia and Nell both nodded.

Before the 9:00 a.m. orientation, the four lined up at the registrar's office to pick up class schedules. On the way to the auditorium for orientation, Ida studied the typed list. "My clinics overlap two of my classes. I don't understand. Cornell wrote that I had a deficit in clinic hours, but I didn't anticipate missing classes."

"Mine is the same," Nell said. "How are we going to keep up?"

"We're going to have to rely on our books and not the class lectures to pass," Margaret said.

"When orientation is over, let's compare schedules. Surely we won't all be missing class at the same time. We'll take notes for each other," Sylvia said.

When they reached the auditorium, they passed a man outside smoking a cigar. "Doctresses." He tipped his bowler hat.

Ida's temper flared, and she felt her neck heat beneath the high neckline of her dress. "Doctorer." She forced a smile.

"Manners," Nell whispered.

"Either we're all doctors or not," Ida said through gritted teeth as they walked inside.

The auditorium reminded Ida of the operating theater at WMCP. She surveyed the room full of tiered seats. Only a few other women sat among the men. Not as many as she'd hoped to see.

"Are we adventurous?" She pointed to several empty seats in the front row.

"Absolutely," Nell said.

Ida routed a way through the crowded aisle to the front row with the girls behind her.

A rumble started, and Ida turned around and scrutinized the group behind her. Across the auditorium, men stomped their feet and threw kisses. Her friends stood still, looking dazed.

"Oh, blow some kisses back, why don't you?" Ida said to her three friends. She pursed her lips, kissed a palm, and blew a kiss to the auditorium of men. The room erupted in applause.

Ignoring the roar, they sat in the cushioned theater seats. Ida fiddled with her fingers while she waited. Four men approached, dressed in suit jackets and ties. One gentleman led the group. Ida straightened and held the armrests tight.

"Excuse me, ladies. My name is Allan," he said. "May I speak with you a moment?"

"Please do," Ida said, not sure what to expect but doing her best to look composed.

"Welcome to Cornell. My friends and I have been assigned to help your entry into Cornell."

His voice sounded kind and Ida relaxed her grip on the armrest.

"I apologize for the men jeering at you," he said.

"I see it as good-natured fun," Ida said, watching her friends who nodded.

"Nevertheless, each one of us is committed to smoothing the transition into academia with the male species." Allan ran his hand across his jaw. "Not every gentleman here has accepted your entrance into their world."

The gentleman motioned for the men behind him to step closer. "I'll introduce Ernie, Clyde, and Douglas to you, so you'll recognize them. Our duty includes walking you to classes, the hospital, or confronting any heckling from other men."

Ida, Sylvia, Margaret, and Nell thanked Allan. He bowed and sat in the row behind them.

Now that she was sitting among a sea of men and hearing this gentleman, would her new male classmates create obstacles to stop her? Would they consider her intelligent? Treat her fairly or snub her for being a woman? The worry stung like a mosquito bite.

When orientation finished, Ida, Margaret, Sylvia, and Nell toured the campus with a guide. Classes began the next day on September 1.

Ida rose earlier than ever to study extra every morning. When she missed classes to make up her clinical hours at the hospital, she studied notes from Sylvia,

Margaret, or Nell. And, as Margaret hoped, a few men offered to share their class notes as well.

By spring, Ida, Nell, Sylvia, and Margaret started their maternity residency together. For two weeks, they moved into a room at the Maternity Hospital in downtown New York. Ida set a small suitcase in the corner of the room. Four cots lined the walls.

"This is the most important part of our training. Ever since I left India, all I've wanted to do was to deliver a baby," Ida said.

Ida, Margaret, Sylvia, and Nell, along with thirty male students, met with a hospital nurse and doctor in the hospital supply room reviewing rules and procedures. Metal tables lined the room in rows with surgical tools wrapped in white cloths. One of the supervising doctors explained the contents of the medical bags with everything the residents needed for the in-home visits they were about to conduct in the poorest district of New York City.

The brown leather bags looked more like oversized laundry bags to Ida.

Ida wanted to deliver a baby without a supervising doctor hovering next to her, but could she do it? Apprehension knotted her stomach. She took a deep breath. Of course she could deliver a baby—hopefully not in someone's apartment, but how was that any different than in a zenana in India?

The final weeks of May seemed like one long maze of study, classes, and clinics at the hospital. During her final exam, her eyes felt like shades someone needed to pull down, and she blinked constantly to stay awake. Numb from the final push to complete school, graduation seemed like another assignment.

After their final test, Ida, Margaret, Sylvia, and Nell splurged on a fancy dinner in downtown New

York City to celebrate and spend one last evening together. They chatted, laughed, and reminisced until nightfall. Ida couldn't imagine taking classes with any better friends than Sylvia, Margaret, and Nell. The next day was busy packing and practicing for graduation.

Graduation morning, as Ida strolled down the aisle to receive her diploma, all she could think was—*seven years of dreaming and is it real? Is this really happening? Am I really a doctor?* Her heart pounded as she heard her name called. "Dr. Ida Scudder."

———

Before leaving for India, Ida worked for the mission to raise funds for a women's hospital in Vellore. After three months of fundraising, contributions weren't near the $8,000 goal. But at the last minute, a widower donated $10,000 for the hospital in honor of his wife—Mary Tabor Schell.

In November Ida boarded the ship for India along with her friend, Annie Hancock, who was also serving as a missionary.

On January 1, 1900, Ida arrived in India knowing God had answered every prayer. Her life was slowly forming a picture.

CHAPTER 25

After reuniting with Father and Marmee, Ida knew she was where she belonged. India was her home. The next day Ida worked alongside her father in the dispensary. But by the end of the first week in Vellore, patients who came to see Father ignored Ida's offer to treat them. She reminded herself several times a day to "wait on the Lord." One by one, each patient refused her. Ida repeated Psalm 27:14 to herself every morning: "Wait on the Lord: be of good courage." Instead of seeing patients as a doctor, side by side with Father she spent the days as his assistant.

Ida and Annie ate lunch each day on the veranda. A woodpecker flittered from branch to branch. Ida wished her life didn't have any cares.

"How are the visits to the zenanas going?" Ida asked.

"Mary Isaac, the missionary training me, and I have visited all thirteen Hindu or Muslim homes who allow Christian visitors. She's moving to work in a remote a village, and I'll minister to the women within Vellore." Annie grinned.

"My work isn't so successful. I haven't examined a single patient yet. I keep reminding myself to wait on the Lord, but patience is not my strongest virtue," Ida said.

"God says to be of good courage." Annie's eyes gleamed, directing them at Ida. "He'll send you patients."

Ida closed her eyes and breathed deeply. "I needed to hear that more than ever. I know this is where God wants me, but the people won't allow me to serve them."

A thud shifted her attention to the road. Ida cupped her ear. A young man ran toward the house.

"Doctor Ammal?" His eyes looked from Ida to Annie.

Ida jumped up and bounced on her feet. "I'm Dr. Scudder."

"My mother . . . she is very sick. Can you help?"

"I'm coming." Ida turned to get her doctor bag. "Wait right here."

He leaned over to catch his breath.

Within moments they were in the carriage on the road to the town center. As the son directed, Souri turned the carriage onto the narrow street toward Fort Hill. When they reached town, Souri parked the wagon on the side of the street.

Ida grabbed her bag and raced behind the young man. The narrow street wound around until they reached a row of houses standing side by side on the edge of the road. She followed him through a huge carved door to the back courtyard. Two rooms opened on either side of a veranda.

The moment Ida ran into the courtyard, children dropped their toys. Women abandoned their bowls of spices beside a grinding stone. A fuchsia-colored sari billowed from behind a column where an old woman crouched.

The young man spoke to the woman behind the column. He spoke so fast Ida didn't understand him, but the woman came out from behind the pillar and led Ida to a dark room. Ida held the wall as she made her way to a heap in the back. The thick tropical air in the room clamped around Ida like a vice. No window. No light. The room was more like a prison than a bedroom. After her eyes adjusted to the darkness, she found a woman lying on a mat on the ground.

The patient lay on her side, curled into a ball of pain, her back to Ida. She bent beside her patient and slid the gold bangles on her arm upward. Her skin was cold. Ida's heart twisted. Was her patient already dead? If the Hindu charmers and self-proclaimed physicians discovered she lost her first patient, her future was doomed. No one would ask for her again.

Ida rubbed the patient's dry skin and pressed her fingers on her wrist. The pulse was faint. The family had waited too late to call a doctor. The young man waited at the entryway, and Ida turned toward him. "Your mother will not live long."

His face crinkled into sudden grief. "No hope?"

"There is nothing I can do to save her." Saying those words wrenched her heart. Saving women's lives was what she'd trained to do. Ida stared at the son for his reaction.

Tears flooded his eyes.

"I will make her comfortable until . . ." Ida didn't want to finish the sentence. Telling him there was no hope was so hard.

The man clapped. Three women sulked from behind tall columns. "Wives, do anything Doctor Missy says."

The women stood as silent and still as the pillars in the courtyard.

"I need her moved out of this stifling room." Ida pointed to a covered spot on the veranda. "Please take her to the shade. If I can't save her, at least she'll be comfortable."

The women carried the patient out and set her beside a shade tree where Ida waited.

The patient's parched and swollen lips were obvious in the sunlight.

"I need a *kuja*, a jar of water," Ida said.

The women grimaced and clenched their saris with their fists. "You moved her to the light. Water is not good for the sick," the oldest woman said. "Are you trying to kill her?"

"Do what the doctor says," the son yelled.

Silently, they filled a jar from the well in the courtyard.

Ida carefully poured water into a brass goblet and spooned water into the woman's mouth. Rinsing a handkerchief and squeezing the excess water out, she bathed her patient, starting with her arms, neck, and forehead.

Before Ida finished bathing, the patient opened her eyes. Ida smiled. "I hope you feel better." From the corner of her eye, Ida could see the patient's eyes tracking her movements. Tenderly, Ida wet the parched skin, humming a hymn while she worked, hoping the feeble efforts would help.

Ten minutes later some of the other women and children came out of hiding. One child squatted next to Ida and held Ida's hand.

Ida gulped. One tiny hand warming her right hand, another cold, withered hand in her left. She blinked back tears.

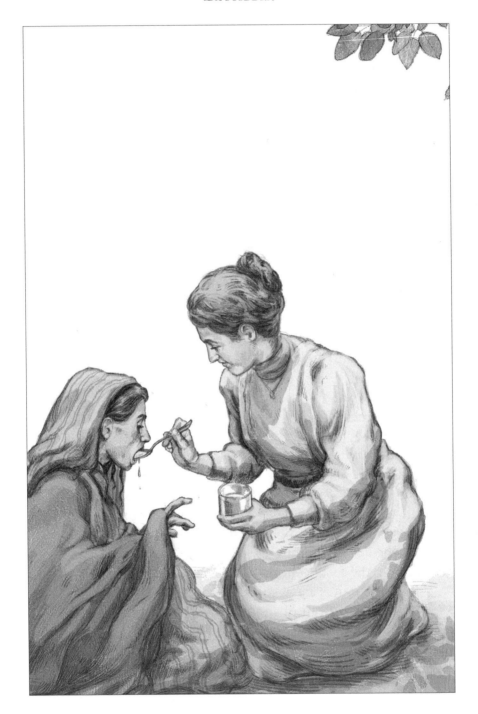

Ida stayed with her patient for the rest of the afternoon, checking vital signs every thirty minutes. Late afternoon shadows spread palm frond shapes across the courtyard. When the old woman's arms stiffened, Ida couldn't watch any longer. She gathered her medical bag and stood.

The patient stirred and began to pull herself along the ground.

"*Illai.* No." Ida screamed.

She continued to crawl toward Ida.

"Don't use your energy—"

With one last push the woman reached Ida, kissed the top of her feet, then dropped her head to the ground.

Ida's throat choked. She bent, checked her pulse. *Why did she use her last bit of strength on me?* "I'm sorry," Ida said to the son. Gently she closed the woman's eyelids.

The daughters-in-law whimpered.

The son hovered over his mother's body. "No!" he wailed.

Ida fumbled out of the courtyard through the narrow path. Before she reached the carriage, the cries echoed off the walls along the road leading back to town. When word traveled, the Hindu families would reject her.

Ida fumbled back into the carriage. *I'm a failure. Everything I've worked for is a waste—my education, Mr. Schell's gift for the hospital. Why did I think I could save women's lives?*

Clouds covered the setting sun. The drum sounded the woman's death message. No one would trust her now.

CHAPTER 26

Within a month, however, some patients did accept Ida as she worked alongside her father in the dispensary. But six months later, her father died. In spite of the emotional setback, Ida didn't give up. Gradually more and more women came to Ida with their medical needs. Within two years, the Mary Tabor Schell Memorial Hospital opened.

By 1903 another doctor, Dr. Louisa Hart, joined the hospital staff. Ida decided to visit patients in the villages surrounding Vellore. Helping people who couldn't reach the hospital excited Ida. Naming their weekly trips "Roadside," Ida packed suitcases of medicine and equipment, took the train to Gudiyattam, twenty miles away, and hired a jutka to drive into the villages every Wednesday. Not every village accepted her. In Lathery the women called her "polluted," but one week on her way through Lathery, a group of men approached her with a bullock.

"My bullock is sick," the owner said. "Will you make it well?"

"I will see what I can do," Ida said. She understood a bullock was as important as a member of the family. Without a bullock they couldn't farm or travel. Ida stepped beside the animal, but it stamped and kicked.

Ida jerked back. "Your bullock isn't going to allow me to touch her."

Men in the village gathered around the bullock, pushed it to the ground, and sat on it while Ida examined the animal.

Ida removed a tumor from the bullock's ear, cleaned her instruments, and left. When she stopped in Lathery the next week, she wondered if the bullock was alive. If her medical treatment killed their bullock, they might come after her.

One of the village elders waited on the side of the road for Ida and shared the good news when she asked. "Yes, the bullock recovered, and the village of Lathery is accepting Dr. Ida's treatments."

———————

The next year the hospital overflowed. After she opened extra beds on the hospital veranda, she wrote the mission headquarters to request an expansion for the hospital. The mission agreed and sent money to make M. T. Schell a sixty-seven-bed hospital. As soon as the hospital enlarged, Ida could see the expansion wasn't enough. Vellore needed a new hospital, more trained staff, and a car to reach more villages.

One morning at church Ida sang with the rest of the congregation, "Be Thou My Vision." Ida prayed God's vision was what she was seeing in her mind. What Vellore really needed was for the Indian women to learn to help themselves. Why not train the local girls as certified nurses? Why wait for the mission to send nurses from other places when she had a community of women surrounding her? After the service, Ida wrote the mission board for permission to begin a school of nursing.

In 1906, Ida left with Marmee for her first furlough to the United States and traveled to Nebraska to her brother Lew's farm for a family reunion. Ida was thrilled to be around her brothers, their wives, and nieces and nephews, especially her seven-year-old namesake, Ida Belle Scudder.

During the two-year furlough, Ida spoke to church audiences and mission meetings whenever she could. One by one, groups contributed money to the mission for a school of nursing.

In 1908, thirty-eight-year-old Ida returned to Vellore with enough money to turn her dream into a reality.

CHAPTER 27

1909

Ida and Marmee arrived home from furlough along with a new car, packed by sections in a crate. Ida hired a mechanic in Madras to put the car together. The night before Ida's first Roadside trip since returning from furlough, Ida and her driver, Roger, loaded the new Peugeot with bedding, folding tables, boxes and bags of medical supplies, medicine, and water jugs.

Roger pushed the folding top onto the back of the one-cylinder Peugeot, loaded the boxes in the floorboards, and tied the last of the supplies everywhere. He peered into the packed car. "There's hardly room for you to sit." He laughed.

"Think of how many more villages I can reach now." Ida crossed her arms and gave a deep, satisfying sigh. "This is progress."

The next morning Ida, Roger, Salomi, and a Bible teacher drove through Vellore to the villages. The car belched black smoke and huffed as if it had a case of bronchitis. After hearing the noisy engine, Ida knew the car wouldn't need an announcement upon their arrival in Vellore.

When Roger honked the horn, bullock carts, cows, and bicyclists, and pedestrians scrambled off the roads. The villagers who lived along the road ran into the fields.

"The devil is coming!" someone screamed.

At their first stop, no one waited for Ida beneath the normal meeting spot, a shady banyan tree off the roadside.

"They're afraid," Ida said. "They don't know what a car is." She turned toward the villages. "We've got to walk to the villages and treat patients. There I can explain the car to them."

The crew carried supplies in their arms and walked. Everyone hid until a naked boy came to Ida, holding his ear. "I have a rock in my ear. Can doctor get it out?"

Ida took her scope and looked in his ear canal. "I can remove the stone, but it might hurt. Are you brave?"

He nodded, and Ida helped him climb onto the examination table that Roger had set up beneath the banyan tree.

"How did you get a stone in your ear?"

"A friend pushed the rock in." He shut his eyes tight but didn't wince while Ida worked on his ear. When she finished, he smiled, and jumped from the table to the ground.

Ida rummaged through a box of postcards and held one out for him. "This is a car. It makes a loud noise, but it's a bullock cart without the bullock. I rode one today. Did you hear it?"

"Yes." His teeth gleamed against his cocoa-colored skin.

"When I leave, walk back to the road with me, and I'll let you honk the horn."

The little boy ran off and came back a minute later holding another boy's hand. "He has a rock in his ear too."

Ida helped his little friend to the table. The area around his ear looked as red as his tearing eyes.

The boy stood next to his friend. "Don't worry. Doctor won't hurt you any more than she has to." He handed the card to his friend. "You can see her car when she's done."

When Ida completed the stone removal, each boy held a coin in the air. "Where is the charity box?"

Salomi held the box toward them, and each one dropped a *pie*, a coin worth one-sixteenth of a cent, in the box.

After the boys, two villagers crept out of their huts to see Ida. Gradually a line formed with people holding coconut shells, flower vases, and empty bottles to hold their medicine. Within a couple of hours, Ida treated forty patients.

When they drove to the next village, people threw stones at the car until a man in the crowd yelled, "The doctor gives medicine to people who are sick. *Pavum!* Shame on anyone who throws stones."

Ida watched them drop their stones while the man who'd admonished them came to Ida and showed her his injured arm. Soon every bystander formed a line.

Miles up the road, children gathered under a shade tree, some standing and some squatting. Some wore loin cloths and others nothing at all.

After ordering her driver to stop, Ida stepped from the car and greeted the children.

The children backed away. Their eyes looked swollen, crusty, and oozing.

"Salomi, I need picture cards, please. Every child here has conjunctivitis."

Ida squatted and held the colored picture until a girl came over to see the card. "Can I look at your eyes?" Ida said. "I will give you medicine to make your eyes better."

The girl clasped her hands in front of her. "Yes."

Ida put the card in the girl's hand, administered drops in both her eyes, and motioned for another child.

"Stop." A bony-looking man from the village ran at Ida, cursing and threatening her in his native tongue.

Ida pointed to the car. "He's angry. We've got to leave."

The crew sped away to the next village. By the end of the day, Ida had visited ten villages. She treated dysentery, guinea worm, scabies, leprosy, and many with conjunctivitis, cataracts, and blindness. It was near dusk when the crew started their trek back to Vellore. Ida saw the glow of tiny lights from lanterns. A man stood in the road waving his hand.

"Don't stop," Ida said to Roger. "I am too exhausted." She'd been on the road since 6:30 a.m. Louisa Hart was on furlough. One doctor wasn't enough to meet the needs of everyone. When would the mission send another doctor? If they sent a dozen, it wouldn't be enough.

Roger swerved the car past the man.

She watched the man run after the car. "Stop, I changed my mind. I must help."

"We need to keep going," Roger said above the noise of the engine. "It is late."

"I can't turn my back on anyone in need."

Roger braked and Ida stepped out. "*Yenna?* What do you need?" She recognized the same man who had chased her that morning. Her heart skipped. Was he going to hurt her?

The man bowed; the tail of his turban trailed in the dirt. "Doctor Ammal." He beckoned the little girl she'd treated that morning, and she came and stood in front of Ida. "Her eyes are better, and we have many children with sore eyes. Would you be kind enough to give us more magic medicine?"

Ida smiled. Another miracle.

CHAPTER 28

In 1911, Ida and Marmee spent May and June in Kodaikanal. Besides rest and recreation, Ida attended the annual Kodaikanal Missionary Medical Conference. Ida's mind buzzed like a bee flirting with a flower garden. Should she share her idea or wait?

During one of the many meetings, Ida sat beside two colleagues, Dr. Anna Kugler and Dr. McPhail, at a large table. From the open window, the scent of eucalyptus wafted in. The mountain peaks reminded her of God's Word; faith could move mountains. Nothing was impossible for God. Encouraged, she looked around the room at the thirty other doctors. Ida decided waiting for another time to propose a medical school in Vellore was not the right direction. Why wait?

Ida raised her hand for a turn to speak during open discussion. She got straight to her point. "In the United States, the average doctor serves six hundred patients. In India, there are a ten thousand patients for every doctor. We need more doctors in India."

The doctors clapped.

"I propose we start a medical school for women in south India immediately."

"Why, the cost is prohibitive," the doctor with a twitchy mustache said.

An older doctor harrumphed. "The mission boards would not agree."

Ida felt a flush rise up her neck. Why had she rushed to speak?

"Ida, there are seven medical schools for men in India." Her cousin Lew gave her a mournful look.

Ida's skin tingled and blood pounded in her ears. She hadn't prepared herself for a betrayal. Not even her cousin understood. He knew the plight of women in India. She thought she'd at least have Lew's support. Ida took a deep breath and said a silent prayer. Too many more negative comments could kill this idea.

"Impossible," shouted a doctor from the back.

Ida didn't recognize the doctor. If only she could escort him and his negative voice out. She scooted in her chair, wishing she'd waited. Why hadn't she talked individually to doctors instead of approaching the entire troop at once? One conversation at a time would have been less embarrassing than facing an army of opponents.

"I support the idea," Dr. Kugler said. "I've dreamt of building a medical school for women too." She tilted her head toward Ida and smiled.

Finally someone agreed. Ida's pulse drummed against her neck. Her hands broke out in a sweat. She wanted to clap. Instead she slid her palms across her skirt, trying to look calm.

"I suggest we appoint a committee to study the project," Dr. McPhail said.

Ida pressed her fingers against her smile. She had two supporters out of a roomful of negatives. She must convince everyone. "We represent a variety of denominations, but we can all agree on one idea." She looked around the room and made eye contact with the audience. "We are building God's kingdom, not a school."

After a long discussion, the doctors agreed to form a committee. "In May 1912, at our annual meeting next year," Dr. McPhail said, "the committee will report on the feasibility of a women's medical college in southern India."

CHAPTER 29

1912–1919

The next year the committee approved a medical college for women. Now Ida needed to launch another fundraiser to build the school. She had already picked out two hundred acres in Vellore for the college, and after a four year wait the Governor of Madras purchased the land for the school. Ida spent her furlough in the United States fundraising and returned with only twenty-five percent of the funds they needed.

Five years passed, and the medical college still had not opened. They owned land, but needed more money to build. When Ida got impatient, Marmee reminded her, "Even God takes His time to grow a tree."

By 1917, Ida decided how to open a medical school without a bigger hospital or additional buildings. Early one morning, she boarded the train for a day trip to Madras. The train blurred past the rice fields. A family of workers waded through the paddies, digging, and planting in the muddy water. In five months, the farmers would harvest the rice. Ida wished progress around the hospital moved as fast as the growing season.

Three hours later Ida arrived in Madras and hired a jutka cart to take her to the government hospital. With the exception of the cows and bullock carts, Madras looked more like a modern American city than Vellore.

The city churches chimed eleven o'clock as she entered the hospital. She knew God would take care of the building needs at the right time. M. T. Schell Hospital was growing. Beginning a medical school was the only wish she needed Colonel Bryson to grant today.

Ida straightened her dress, climbed the stairs, and knocked on the office door for Colonel Bryson, the director of the British Medical Department. The door swung open and his mustached lips spread in a wide grin. "What an honor to have a visit from the Dr. Ida." Colonel Bryson pulled a chair out for Ida and slid a rattan-backed chair for himself beside her.

The office was furnished in rich mahogany, framed diplomas, and a silver tea set on the tea table beside the window. Outside, a palm brushed a frond against the window as the breeze ruffled the bottom of Ida's dress.

"What is on your mind?" Colonel Bryson leaned forward, clasping his hands on his lap. "I know you're not here for chitchat."

Ida chuckled. "I'd like approval to begin a medical school for women in Vellore to earn their Licensed Practitioner Diploma." Her heart hammered against her chest. She sat erect and kept her hands clasped. She hoped Colonel Bryson couldn't see how nervous she really was.

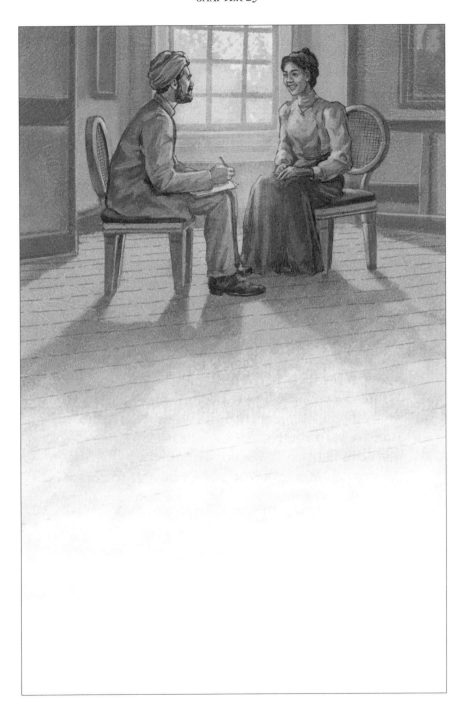

He grinned and leaned back. "You traveled eighty miles to make a joke?"

"I'm serious. We'll raise our standards to gain university affiliation as we grow." She paused and smiled. "I need the approval of your office to open the school."

Colonel Bryson cleared his throat. "Do you have a building? Do you have money?"

"I'll rent buildings near the hospital until we build. I'll teach all the medical classes. Our students will take physics and chemistry at the local college, Voorhees College."

Colonel Bryson lost the amused look on his face. "A school of medicine for Indian women?"

Ida bristled inside. She hadn't expected the conversation to be an easy one. She squared her shoulders. "Colonel Bryson, is the hospital in Madras lacking medical doctors as mine is?" She smiled, confidence running through her. He couldn't deny the need. "Train the people who live here to work here."

"Are you prepared to send these women to the exams and to compete against the men?" He smirked. "The competition is steep."

"Are you afraid the men won't be able to compete with the Indian women?" Ida flashed him a playful grin.

He laughed and shook his head. "I seriously doubt you'll get three applicants. However, if you can secure six applicants, you have government permission."

Ida restrained herself from hugging him and said, "Thank you, Colonel Bryson. I'll have the six applicants needed."

Her feet bounced off the floor. She was going to throw herself into work. Happy tears seeped from her eyes.

A week later Ida stuffed envelopes with the announcement—"A Medical School for Women is to be opened in July 1918 in Vellore"—and included the application, mailing them to every girls' school surrounding Vellore. Over the next two months Ida visited mission and government schools, recruiting and interviewing candidates for the women's medical school.

Sixty-nine applications arrived with one addressed to *Empty Shell* Hospital instead of *M. T. Schell.* She selected eighteen students, a mix of Hindu, Muslim, and Christian girls, and sent each a letter of congratulations and instructions for the opening.

Ida rose each day at 3:00 a.m. to prepare for classes with the limited equipment she owned—one skeleton, one microscope, and two text books. The students started each day at morning chapel. Ida began every Monday by reading from 1 Corinthians 13 to show the students how to treat their patients with love. Even among the different belief systems of her girls, Ida believed the most important thing she could teach was God's love.

The girls often ate meals together with Ida at her bungalow or at the medical students' bungalow. Occasionally Ida packed a picnic and gave the girls a break from studying. Ida attended social gatherings only if her students also were invited.

As the first year ended in March and the yearly doctor's test in Madras approached, Ida started to second guess herself. Did she have enough equipment to prepare her girls? Did she test them enough? The day of the test, Ida and her class took the train to the Madras Medical Department. Her stomach roiled as she escorted them to the classroom, more nervous than when she took her own medical exams.

"Do your best." She grinned in spite of the terror pumping through her. "The test won't be any worse than my quizzes." The Madras Medical School intimidated her with its well-stocked library, models of organs, and numerous skeletons for the students to study. Why had she been so sure she could teach? And with one skeleton? *Dear God, the outcome of my students is up to you. Please help them remember what they've learned.*

Ida smiled at Colonel Bryson when she stopped him in the hallway, making sure he couldn't read her last-minute panic.

"Dr. Ida." Colonel Bryson looked pleased to see her. "Don't be upset if your girls don't pass. The exam is stiff. Only twenty percent of the men pass. I'm behind your school, so don't give up." His cheeks dimpled when he smiled.

Ida stood a little taller. "My girls worked hard over the past year. They're prepared for this exam."

Back in Vellore five days later, Colonel Bryson arrived at Ida's bungalow. "I wanted to bring the students' scores to you in person."

Ida wasn't sure if seeing Colonel Bryson was good news or bad news. "A visit from you is an honor." Her heart raced like stampeding cattle.

Shaking, she opened the envelope and scanned the page.

"As I told you," Colonel Bryson said, "only one out of five men passed. I'm afraid your girls are setting a difficult standard for the men."

"Excuse me, Colonel Bryson." Clutching the note, she ran from the bungalow to the girls' bungalow, screaming, "Ladies! Every one of you passed your first year of medical school."

The girls congregated around Ida while she took each one in her arms, laughing and crying.

CHAPTER 30

1920–1930

By the next school year, two hundred girls applied to the medical school. Ida wanted to say yes to every qualified candidate, but M. T. Schell Hospital was too small. To increase the size of the school, the hospital needed more beds to meet the government requirements of three patient beds per medical student.

When Ida wasn't teaching or caring for patients, she campaigned to raise money for the hospital and school. Construction for a new hospital, dispensary, and nurses' housing began in 1921.

Ida's first class of medical students graduated on March 22, 1922, with their Licensed Medical Practitioner Diplomas. Colonel Bryson addressed the crowd for the convocation. "Dr. Ida Scudder took on a daring project, and today we see the results of the past four years. My skepticism turned to admiration after I witnessed Ida's close relationship with her students."

Ida thought of the hours and hours of demanding work for her girls, for her doctors, feeling as proud and joyful as if she were their mother. She remembered the reason she studied medicine—to serve mothers in need. Now a group of women had followed the call to serve women in India.

At the sound of the applause, Ida stood to hand diplomas to these new doctors.

She smiled to herself, knowing that with God nothing was impossible.

EPILOGUE

During her lifetime, Ida met the famous minister and author, Norman Vincent Peale, enjoyed tea at the White House with First Lady, Mrs. Roosevelt, and hosted a visit from Mahatma Gandhi and numerous dignitaries throughout India. She was awarded the Kaisar-i-Hind Medal for Public Service and the Award of Distinction from Cornell University Alumni Association. After fifty years of service and for Ida's golden eightieth birthday, the citizens of Vellore raised the money to build a new road—the Dr. Ida Scudder Road.

On May 24, 1960, Ida died at her home at the age of eighty-nine.

As Ida had hoped, the hospital expanded. Today Vellore is one of the largest hospital systems in India. Christian Medical College and Hospital ranks among the most distinguished medical institutions in India. Both the hospital and college continue to make a difference in people's lives by treating patients with the same attitude Ida established—to witness God's healing power through education, research, and service.

TERMS

ammal: woman, mother, matron

bindi: a colored dot worn in the middle of the forehead, usually worn by Hindu women

bullock: ox

chapati: flat bread

chota: morning coffee and bread or small breakfast

congee: a rice porridge

dhobi: washerman

ghee: clarified butter

godown: a warehouse

illai: no

jutka: a one-horse carriage with a canopy

palanquin: a large, covered box on poles carried by bearers to transport people

pferd: German word for horse

pukka: Hindu word for permanent

sari: a length of cotton or silk that is wrapped around a woman's waist, shoulders, and head

tamarind: a tree

tamil: language spoken in Indian State of Tamil Nadu

zenana: woman's private living area in an Indian home